SPARK N FLY

The 5 Pillars for Taking Control of Your Health

Isabelle Paquette

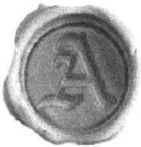

AuthoritiesPress

SPARK N FLY: The 5 Pillars for Taking Control of Your Health
www.sparknflynow.com

Copyright © 2018 Isabelle Paquette

ISBN-13: 978-1772772265 (10-10-10 Publishing)
ISBN-10: 1772772267

Limits of Liability and Disclaimer of Warranty
The author and publisher shall not be liable for your misuse of the enclosed material. This book is strictly for informational and educational purposes only.

Warning – Disclaimer
The purpose of this book is to educate and entertain. The author and/or publisher do not guarantee that anyone following these techniques, suggestions, tips, ideas, or strategies will become successful. The author and/or publisher shall have neither liability nor responsibility to anyone with respect to any loss or damage caused, or alleged to be caused, directly or indirectly by the information contained in this book.

Medical Disclaimer
The information within this book is not intended or implied to be a substitute for professional medical advice, diagnosis or treatment regarding the readers health. All content, including text, graphics, images and information, contained within this book and website is for general information purposes only. The author/publisher makes no representation and assumes no responsibility for the accuracy of information contained on or available within this book and through the website, and such information is subject to change without notice. You are encouraged to confirm any information obtained within this book or through the website with other sources and review all information regarding any medical condition or treatment with your physician. NEVER DISREGARD PROFESSIONAL MEDICAL ADVICE OR DELAY SEEKING MEDICAL TREATMENT BECAUSE OF SOMETHING YOU HAVE READ ON OR ACCESSED.

Publisher
10-10-10 Publishing
Markham, ON Canada

Printed in Canada and the United States of America

TABLE OF CONTENTS

Dedication

To my Creator God, who inspired me to go head first into life and to live intensely and fully until my last breath.

ACKNOWLEDGEMENTS

The writing of this book was dotted with hardships. It was a therapy for me, a way to escape by putting on paper the knowledge that I have accumulated over time.

Cancer, and the many surgeries of my former life partner, made me grow, and made me discover the woman in me, who has such a great need to share and impact the lives of the people around her. My greatest reward is to see, hear, and especially feel the gratitude of people who have improved their health and quality of life by following my advice on the management of the 5 pillars of health. I thank *Mario Pilon* for being a very important person in my life. You allowed me to reinforce my belief in my life mission, which is to help people make better choices that realign them to true health. You also led me to create this vision of an epidemic of healthy people around the world. I send you love, joy, happiness, gratitude, healing, and the most important, faith. May God take care of you and guide you to your life mission.

I thank *my family*, who are slowly opening up to health. I have always hoped to see you taking care of yourselves and opting for health.

I thank *my colleagues, my partners,* and especially all those who work near me and who are part of my team. Your support and your faith in my mission lead me to always push the limits of the impossible. Together, we are working to make a real difference in people's lives in terms of their physical, mental, emotional, and financial health. A special mention to Serge Deslongchamps and Diane Monette Deslongchamps, who have always supported me and who have always believed in my abilities.

My friends:

I thank my true friends, who have always been there for me and have supported me in difficult times. Marie-Lou Kerr, Carine Goyette, Vickie Hébert, and Cathy Melvin, you are wonderful friends! Jason Fuoco, who was only a young child when I taught him taekwondo, and today he is a friend I can really rely on. Van Quan Phung, who has been here since our first meeting in martial arts. Jimmy Girard, a friend and almost fraternal brother, with whom I built my strength and speed in taekwondo, because you were my faithful and talented training partner. Robert Berger, a friend, who was able to give me a hand in the English-language correction of my book. Yves Dugré, a friend who has always believed in me and in my potential. Your spirituality and your need to contribute to this world have had an impact in my life.

Finally, to all my friends, who shared and crossed my path. Know that you are all important!

My Taekwondo world:

Grand Master Chong Lee, who left this world on July 5, 2017, and who brought to the world of martial arts (taekwondo) an exceptional level of knowledge. I had the privilege of receiving your lessons, and even your coaching, at the world championships. Master Christian Sourdif, who taught me from the age of 7, and saw me grow and evolve in this magnificent martial art that is taekwondo.

To *my clients,* who have always believed in me and have given me their full confidence.

Finally, to *my publishing team,* who believed in me and who were very patient. Liz Ventrella, who guided me through the steps and made sure that each piece was in place at the right time. Tracy Knepple, who worked with me to ensure that the chapters were well formulated.

To *Raymond Aaron*, who encouraged me to write my book, for the first time at an event in Orlando, and who believed in me.

FOREWORD

Isabelle Paquette has an amazing ability to recognize how critical your health is in your ability to live a life of purpose and passion. In *Spark N Fly*, Isabelle takes you on a journey through the common health beliefs, identifying the truth about what you eat, and how it impacts your health.

Isabelle spells out the 5 pillars and ties each one to creating an epidemic of healthy people, while outlining how you can be one of them. Her clear and precise explanations allow you to see how to apply these steps in every aspect of your life, allowing you to move forward with clarity and purpose.

Right from chapter one, Isabelle gives you the tools to understand the labels on food and supplements, before moving into how you can become healthy in all areas of your life beyond the physical.

If you are ready to get healthy, then I encourage you to pick up *Spark N Fly*, and take flight to the healthiest you can be!

Raymond Aaron
New York Times Bestselling Author

INTRODUCTION
A Health Crisis in the Making

I have been in the health field since 2004. My previous career as a physiotherapist, and my present career as an osteopath, have permitted me to observe firsthand the recurring problems of my clients. During my discussions with these clients, I have noticed a pattern of health problems that are related to the digestive system. These problems encompass a variety of issues, such as chronic constipation, diarrhea, irritable bowel, Crohn's disease, ulcerative colitis, colon cancer, gastric reflux and stomach burning, difficulty digesting certain foods, swelling, bloating, and flatulence—and the list could go on.

There is also a significant increase in degenerative diseases globally. Cancer, diabetes, strokes, Alzheimer's disease, fibromyalgia, osteoporosis, osteoarthritis, cardiovascular diseases, and depression have continued to take their toll, despite medical advancements meant to halt their progression. How do we address most of these diseases and health issues? Unfortunately for us, we are being taught to address these issues at the pharmacy counter.

As an osteopath and a naturopath, I feel privileged because I maintain a special relationship with my clients. Sometimes I see clients only once a year, only to find out that they are still taking medication. But are these medications the cure, or just another part of a larger health crisis? The answer appears to be related to changes in our environment.

Realities and Our Toxic Environment

The environment in which we live is not the same one our grandparents grew up in. For example, carrots would turn your hand slightly orange as you peeled them. Today, that is no longer the case. Beta-carotene used to be present in large amounts, hence the reason your hands turned orange, but it appears to be missing from carrots today. This vitamin is critical, not only for the health of our eyes, but also to prevent certain cancers, diabetes, Alzheimer's disease, headache, high blood pressure, infertility, and skin disorders. What is prompting the changes in our food supply?

The land used for farming has been exploited, denatured, and drained of nutrients over time. If these essential nutrients are not in the earth, then how can they make it into our fruits and vegetables? In addition to the lack of nutrients, humans have introduced pollution, pesticides, and other potentially toxic chemicals into the water, air, and earth.

How much time do you think passes between picking and actually eating fruits? The process of getting our food into our hands often comes at a cost. Here's just a few of the steps from the fields to our dinner tables:

- Picking (local, national, and international)
- Transportation to the grocery store
- Storage
- Exhibition in grocery shelves
- Purchase of food
- Fridge, congelation
- Baking (often high temperature)

What nutrients remain after such a long period between when your food was on the vine or in a tree, and when you actually get to eat it? This situation makes it hard to get everything your body needs, in a non-toxic fashion, from food alone.

In fact, I would say that it is IMPOSSIBLE to find all the nutrients in foods that we need for our cells to protect our bodies from the myriad of health issues and diseases around today. Scientific studies have shown us that we lose large quantities of nutrients (vitamins and minerals) in our foods in the present! These studies show us that certain vitamins and certain minerals are practically non-existent or at quite small levels in our foods.

Eating Well? Not Likely!

People eat poorly, often relying on processed foods for their nutritional needs. Many individuals believe they eat well, when in fact, it's quite the opposite! In my office, when I ask clients if they eat well, the answer is almost always yes. That is until we start discussing what they are eating daily. These forays into their daily diets have shown me that most individuals do not know what to eat or how to prepare it to maximize their nutritional benefits.

Thus, it is important to look at the people and businesses in our society that benefit from this lack of knowledge and the health issues that can often result. Who should claim some responsibility?

Providing Disease Insurance : The Medical Industry

When you stop to think about it, the medical industry is the only one where increases in illness can actually be good for business. In Canada, we pay for a public health insurance system with our tax returns. In the United States, it's a private health insurance. Therefore, the more visits we have, the more money they make. That does not provide incentive for a doctor to find the source of your symptoms but can motivate them to only focus on treating your symptoms. No prevention!!!

Then we must look at the pharmaceutical companies. A need for profits drives their business model, so they encourage doctors to prescribe medication for a variety of illnesses. These companies are not seeking to help individuals, as much as they are looking to line their pockets. Hence, the lack of research on diseases that are rare, because they are simply less profitable in the long run. Therefore, it is in their best interests to lobby the government for regulations that are favorable to them, often at the expense of the patients' interests. **Cures are simply not good business!**

Neither is attempting to find the source of health issues or diseases. Studies that explore how and why we get cancer, for instance, involve finding more expensive tests and more drugs, without necessarily determining ways to avoid cancer altogether. Other diseases, such as diabetes, obesity, cardiovascular disease, fibromyalgia, and digestive problems, suffer the same fate. The reason is simple. Healthy people do not visit the doctor, and they do not have to fill prescriptions. Hence, they do not contribute to the bottom line of the medical industry.

DISEASES AND SYMPTOMS = $$$
HEALTH = No Money

What are the alternatives to the traditional medical industry and its methods? Let's find out!

Taking Control of Your Health

My experiences have shown me that true health can be achieved, and the more individuals who achieve this healthy state, the more we can create global health. So how is it possible to get healthy and stay that way?

Several areas need to be addressed to create a healthy lifestyle, both now and throughout your life. By addressing these areas with the tools provided in this book, you can regain your health, as well as see an increase in your energy level. Yes, you can be part of a global health epidemic!

Finding Health with Wisdom

Knowledge and wisdom assist us in making the right decisions. Without this combination, you are lost and can make bad choices that will impact your life. Therefore, it is critical to invest the time to gain knowledge that you can use to evaluate the soundness of a course of action, hence using wisdom to benefit yourself.

Knowledge and wisdom can put you in the driver's seat regarding your health and wellness. But where can you start to gain both necessary components?

Here are the five pillars of health that will assist you to achieve optimal health:

BODY – MIND – SOCIETY
ENVIRONMENT – FINANCES

MY VISION: CREATING AN EPIDEMIC OF HEALTHY PEOPLE! How can we do this? By sparking our energy and giving our bodies what they need to thrive! Want to join me? Then let's get started!

Pillar 1 :
BODY

Chapter 1

NUTRITIONAL SUPPLEMENTS
ARE A WEAPON!

What Your Cells Need

Your body is composed of 75 to 100 trillion different cells! Organs, bones, cartilage, teeth, soft tissue, skin, and nails are all made from these tiny cells, which also must eat to sustain life. Each cell is like a living organism that must work in harmony with other cells in your body to continuously maintain your health, depending on your lifestyle.

What do your cells actually need? Each of your cells is a factory running 24/7, but the factory cannot produce anything without the raw materials. Your cells are waiting physiologically to get the necessary macronutrients and micronutrients from what you eat daily. Proteins, carbohydrates, fats, and fibers are all macronutrients. The minerals, vitamins, and antioxidants are micronutrients, and where you find the majority of deficiencies.

Nowadays, it is not the MACRONUTRIENTS that are deficient. The only exception is fibers, whose contribution to the health of the body is often ignored. However, fibers have a protective effect in your intestines, in addition to helping your bowels keep everything moving. They also help to reduce your risk of colon cancer, which is the second leading cause of cancer death in Canadian men, and the third leading cause of cancer death in Canadian women, according to the Canadian Cancer Society. In the USA, excluding skin cancers, colorectal cancer is the third most common cancer diagnosed in both men and women, according to American Cancer Society.

The more serious problem is at the MICRONUTRIENT level. For the reasons I mentioned earlier, including overexploited and denatured lands, utilization of pesticides and chemicals agents, transportation, storage, refrigeration, freezing, and baking, you lose those precious nutrients that your cells need to function at their full potential. Maybe you think you have optimal health, but this is because you have never experienced true optimal health!

Here are those essential micronutrients that you need daily. Essential minerals include calcium, magnesium, potassium, phosphorus, zinc, iodine, iron, sodium, boron, silicon, chromium, selenium, etc. There are 13 essential vitamins, which include Vitamin A, Vitamins B1, B2, B3, B5, B6, B8, B9, B12, C, D, E, and K. Don't forget antioxidants, such as bioflavonoids, including quercetin, rutin, hesperidin, resveratrol, green tea, blueberry, pomegranate, cinnamon, and curcumin from turmeric. These act together to inhibit the activity of free radicals. Co-enzyme Q10 and alpha lipoic acid are also so important.

Without the necessary minerals, vitamins, and antioxidants, you're dead! If you are deficient in some of them, your body is not running optimally. Yes, it's IMPOSSIBLE to achieve optimal health without all of them. How does the food industry contribute to the problem of micronutrient deficiencies?

What About the Food Industry?

Almost all the food manufacturers also lie to you, especially when they claim their products are healthy because they have no fat in them. Yes, it's true there is no fat. But what do you think they put in to create that good taste that brings us back to buy their products again and again? They add SUGAR, in larger amounts than most of us realize. Then you eat all this sugar, and your body transforms it into fat! When the manufacturers advertise sugar-free products, they often add a lot of bad fat to make the products tasty without the sugar. They may also add artificial sweeteners! It's not healthy in the short or long term. These are just a few of their tricks. How many more tricks do you think they have?

The most important thing to keep in mind is a healthy dose of skepticism regarding the labels on products. They all advertise products that are healthy, farm fresh, 100%

natural, light, containing omega 3, Vitamin E, and the list goes on. But are all these label listings on a product true? As for the vitamins, do you think they are truly bioavailable? Is it really 100% natural? It's a processed food, so how can it be 100% natural? It doesn't make sense!

The big problem is when you are at the supermarket, you don't want to know where the products originated. You buy whatever is available in front of your eyes. The power of voluntary ignorance is boundless. However, there are still individuals who want to learn about alternatives.

When I coach people, I help them to choose some products to include in their diet that have a good number of good macronutrients. If you have the wrong quantity, it's not going to work. You will not have enough energy to live your life to the fullest!

If it was possible for you to have one meal in your day, where you were sure of the purity, would you take it? I do that every day! I have one meal in my day where I'm sure about the purity, and I know the exact quantity of protein, carbohydrates, and good fat (including coconut oil) that I need. My body is so happy to have all that energy as a result.

The Role of Supplements

For a long time, I studied to find out if it was possible to get these necessary micronutrients by foods alone. I can tell you that it's impossible! Even those of you who eat organic or eat raw will struggle to meet your nutritional needs.

Knowing how important micronutrients are to your cells for you to create optimum health and live an energetic and radiant life, the best way to achieve it is through supplementation.

The role of supplements is to fill in what is missing from your plate! It's simple, right? You are ensuring that your cells have the right food at the right time. By doing this, you optimize your health!

19 Reasons to Supplement

As we have seen, your body runs best when fueled properly. Supplements can assist you in moving in the direction of receiving all that necessary fuel. Here are several more reasons why you need to supplement to address various health concerns, as well as reversing the lack of micronutrients in your system.

1- Soils are depleted by big business agriculture, which includes overproduction, minimal to no crop rotation, no rest for the land, and fertilizer use. Significant loss of minerals, vitamins, and antioxidants in the food is a result.

2- Early picking of fruits and vegetables, especially those from other countries, results in a loss of minerals, vitamins, and antioxidants, as they do not get to ripen on the vine.

3- Transportation from the field to a processing plant, and then to your local store, means that several days have passed. During that time, the fruits and vegetables are losing their nutritional value and can be placed in contact with contaminants. Furthermore, during this process, foods are affected by different temperatures in each location.

4- Food storage occurs in warehouses, refrigerators, and freezers for a period ranging from a few days to weeks, or even months, before being consumed. Thus, there is additional nutrient loss during the storage period.

5- Preparation and cooking is a fact of life. You boil, fry, and cook your food at very high temperatures that destroy micronutrients, but can also create glycotoxins! Using the microwave, according to some research, may even change the molecules of your food.

6- Food allergies and intolerances mean some sources of micronutrients are banished because of allergic or symptomatic reactions to the foods themselves.

7- Special diets often mean you banish certain foods. For example, vegetarian, raw foods, and vegan diets can bring some specific deficiencies. You can see the benefits with some plans on short term. On a long-term basis, specific deficiencies, such as the B12, can cause a variety of problems, including anemia, fatigue, mood problems, and memory loss, even to the point of dementia! You are the result of small choices that have long-term consequences.

8- Food additives, flavors, and artificial colors provide no nutrients. Additionally, processing foods can decrease or even empty them of essential nutrients. Yet processed food is approximately 70% of our food supply.

9- Irradiated food can produce harmful chemicals, in addition to reducing its nutritional content. http://uniondesconsommateurs.ca/docu/agro/irradiatio n_sommex.pdf

10- Chemicals, such as herbicides and pesticides, are used to kill insects and weeds. They have also been added to tap water as part of the filtering process.

11- Other substances and contaminants, which can include heavy metals, petroleum derivatives, hormones, and antibiotics, are found in our food and water. More than 143,000 chemicals have been identified worldwide[1].

12- Drugs may also decrease or prevent the absorption of certain nutrients in our body. For example, coenzyme

Q10 absorption can be interrupted by taking statins, which are prescribed for high cholesterol. Antibiotics are also known to destabilize the intestinal flora.

13- Our lifestyle, including our food choices, our level of physical activity, our various habits (like cigarettes, alcohol, drugs), and even our thoughts, can contribute to less than optimal health, due to the unnecessary stress on our body.

14- Stress can be a powerful destructive force on our body, which can literally draw on our nutrient reserves.

15- When our body is not receiving the proper nutrients, coupled with a lack of sleep or a consistently disrupted sleep cycle, then our body struggles to maintain even a token of health.

16- Various symptoms and diseases are often a sign of a nutritional deficiency. The body then requires more micronutrients to regenerate and repair itself, which further compounds the deficiency.

17- Symptoms of digestive disorders, including digestion problems, difficulty digesting sugars or fats or proteins, heartburn, gastroesophageal reflux, bloating, gas, constipation, diarrhea, stomach aches and abdominal cramps, can all be the result of a lack of the necessary nutrients that should be present in our system to function properly.

18- Joint pain may be due to chronic inflammation and even a sign of certain nutritional deficiencies.

19- Finally, an overall lack of energy can be suggestive of your body's lack of the nutrients it needs to survive and thrive!

As you can see, the list could go on regarding the impact on our systems from a lack of these vital nutrients, which are reduced or missing altogether from our food supply. Because a lot of nutrients are necessary daily, supplements provide a way to guarantee that our body receives them every day in the right quantities. Not receiving them may not show in the short term but can have long term consequences on our overall health. The body is always looking to find a balance. It may be able to manage and compensate for weeks, months, or even years, until it finally reaches the limit and begins to breakdown. Illness then sets in, affecting your life and the lives of your loved ones.

Do you think that cancer suddenly appears?

Vitamin C : Anti-Cancer Agent

Look at how this degenerative disease, CANCER, invades our bodies and our lives. Just the word CANCER can trigger intense feelings of anxiety and fear! There is a good reason for these feelings, as the statistics clearly outline.

This is what awaits us according to the Canadian Cancer Society since June 2017. It is expected that half of Canadians will be diagnosed with cancer at some point in their lives, and that 1 in 4 Canadians will die from this disease. Half of all new cases will be lung, colorectal, breast, and prostate cancers. According to Statistics Canada, in 2011, cancer was the leading cause of disease-related death in children under the age of 15. Do you think the outlook is any better in the USA, or even elsewhere in the world? Certainly not!

According to the World Cancer Report 2014, cancers figure among the leading causes of morbidity and mortality worldwide, with approximately 14 million new cases, and 8.2 million cancer related deaths in 2012[2].

Nobody is safe from this dreadful disease. You may have had cancer or know someone who has dealt with this disease. However, there are weapons to help you, and supplementation is one of them. You should take care of that NOW! Don't wait until you receive a cancer diagnosis. After all, cancers can develop over several years. It is important to make changes as quickly as possible to avert the cancer's growth in your system.

You must also change your mentality that the government will protect you and your health. Governments are invested in rewarding the disease system. You must choose true health and invest in yourself! It's the most powerful gift that you can give to your body and the people that you love. One of the first ways to fight this cancer threat and move toward a healthier you are by increasing your Vitamin C intake. Why?

One of the important vitamins that you can take is VITAMIN C!

According to Dr. Linus Pauling, the foremost authority on Vitamin C, it will decrease your risk of getting certain cancers by 75% if it is consumed on a regular basis. Vitamin C is an antioxidant and enzyme cofactor that can also help to reduce the risk of cardiovascular disease, including coronary heart disease and stroke. However, your body is not able to synthesize and produce vitamin C, like animals can. You must get it from your fruits and vegetables. However, as our discussion has shown, if you are relying on food alone, you will not have enough to protect you from these diseases!

When you look the RDA (Recommended Dietary Allowance), it's so low that you can't protect yourself from disease, because your body does not get enough Vitamin C to be effective! As a safety guideline, the Food and Nutrition Board, Institute of Medicine established a tolerable upper intake level at 2000 mg for Vitamin C in adults[3].

When you take it at that level, you must take bioavailable Vitamin C. It's better to take it at least two times per day because the Vitamin C is a water-soluble vitamin. You will use up your first dose within just a few hours. Still, with two doses a day, you can enjoy the benefits of this vitamin throughout your entire day.

Now, let's move from Vitamin C, a potential protector from cancer and disease, to another critical supplement for your digestive system.

PROBIOTICS : Your Little Soldiers

Farm animals consume approximately 50% of antibiotics produced. These farm animals either produce or become part of the food stock on our dining tables. Those antibiotics are being passed on to you as part of every meal you eat.

Do you know that approximately 70–80% of your immune cells live in your intestines, where you find the critical intestinal flora? Antibiotics destroy your flora, which aids in digestion, assimilation of nutrients, and waste and stool disposal, and is part of your digestive track. When you think about it, the antibiotics in the food supply are destroying your flora, which is necessary for your digestive track to work effectively!

Do you know that doctors often prescribe antibiotics, even if you don't need them? Each time you take them, you are destroying the army that protects you against viruses, bacteria, and various diseases. Logically, if your immune system is weakened, it should be no surprise that you are sick frequently. What do you think happens to people who are on antibiotics for a long period?

If you eat animal products, you probably eat antibiotics. Choose the animal products and meats from manufacturers and farmers that do not use antibiotics. Let's be realistic; we can't check everything. When you go to a restaurant, for example, you will surely have an antibiotic as part of your meal.

But it's not only the antibiotics that are problematic. What else could affect the flora in your intestines? Stress, chemical agents, food additives, processed foods, medication, and the list could go on. When you add everything together, it's a destructive cocktail.

WHAT CAN YOU DO TO PROTECT YOUR IMMUNE SYSTEM AND INTESTINAL FLORA?

The best defense is a good offense. In this case, you must take a supplement of **PROBIOTICS** to protect you. But most of the probiotics on the market are a poor-quality option. There are so many ads on TV for these supplements because the manufacturers know that you need them with the foods available and the frequent exposure to antibiotics. It's very important to have a probiotic that will pass the stomach acid barrier to get to the main target: your intestines. Most of the supplements that you see on TV do almost nothing. They put probiotics with yogurt, milk, cheese, and soya, and then they add sugar to make it taste good.

In the end, the probiotics don't play their role, because they never make it out of the stomach. So, when you are looking for a probiotics supplement, you must be sure the sources of bacteria can survive passage through the stomach and influence the intestinal flora to promote digestive health and immune function. It's time to take action. Spark your digestive system with a quality probiotic supplement, and you will soar toward a healthier you! SPARK N FLY!

It's not ONLY about the quantities of the bacteria but the quality. Without viable bacteria, the effects will be minimal on your digestive health.

Swim in Essential Fatty Acids : Omega 3

Have you noticed how omega 3 fatty acids have increased in popularity? Do you know why exactly? The food industry knows, and that's why it took the opportunity to insert it in many foods (eggs, crackers, cookies, and drinks). But is it bioavailable?

The report in our daily diet of OMEGA 6/OMEGA 3 (O6 / O3) ideally should be around 1/1. The problem is that now we can find reports from 10, 20, 30, and 40 to 1, which puts much more O6 into our systems than we need. When too much is present, then it begins to cause other issues.

When too much O6 is consumed, it synthesizes into prostaglandin of war (PGE2). If the liver gets too much O6, then the liver will transform it into arachidonic acid, the precursor of prostaglandins of war. PGE2 will generate thousands of inflammatory hormones that break the dynamic balance of good health (homeostasis).

The excess of O6 causes inflammatory molecules, and SCIENCE confirms:

INFLAMMATION IS THE SOURCE OF MANY DISEASES!

The level of inflammation within an individual is inversely proportional to their omega 3 circulating levels[4]. High levels of O6 are associated with a risk of cardiovascular diseases, cancers, inflammatory diseases, autoimmune diseases, allergies, athletic performance alterations, and depression, just to name a few.

If you get your omega 3 from fish, you won't get a sufficient amount because you cannot consume fish in mass quantities. Most fish today are full of heavy metals. Thus, you have to limit your servings to 2 or 3 times per week. It is the reason I recommend that my clients take a supplement of omega 3. The supplement helps to balance out the O6/O3 ratio, and can potentially reduce your inflammation as a result.

A nutritional program is incomplete without a high-quality source of omega 3 fatty acids. They must come from fish oils from cold seas, balanced and highly concentrated in two important omega 3 fatty acids, eicosapentaenoic acid (EPA) and docosahexaenoic acid (DHA). Also, it is important that the nutritional supplement of omega 3 holds a *no heavy metals* certification. Most of the companies that make these supplements do not offer this type of certification.

When you choose to supplement, you don't want to find these enemies, such as heavy metals (mercury, aluminum, lead, arsenic), pesticides, petrol, and other contaminants, in your cells because of the supplements you take. Heavy metals are an enemy because of their link with some diseases, including brain diseases, Alzheimer's, loss of memory, and autism, although these are just a few of the potential problems these metals can create.

How can you find the best supplements for your body, which can assist you in joining the epidemic of healthy people?

Most of the Supplements Are Just Scrap!

It's hard to hear, but most supplements available have little to no value. You take them, and they do NOTHING for your system. You take them to increase your health, but the results are simply not there. The manufacturers are lying with misleading labeling. For example, they could say proudly on the label that their products contain 400 UI of vitamin E, but that may not be the case. When you analyze the tablets, each has a different amount of vitamin E. It is even possible to find tablets containing no vitamin E at all. Some of them have such trace amounts of vitamin E that they have no therapeutic value to them. It's just an excellent marketing tactic that ends up lining their pockets. You are thus paying for insufficient vitamin E, and the result is little to no noticeable effect on your body. In poor quality or insufficient quantity, a supplement of vitamin E will do nothing for you and your system.

If that was not bad enough, many supplements also contain ingredients that you do not want in your body but are not included on the label. What are some of these ingredients? Petroleum products, heavy metals, and other contaminants make it into your supplements, and then make their way into your body to cause havoc regarding your quest to join the healthy people epidemic.

How do they get away with it? The primary reason is because no strict standard for supplements to be measured by exists. They can make false allegations or claims, with little to no proof to back them up. Therefore, you should be cautious of supplements sold through television, the Internet, shops, and pharmacies, in part because the supplements may not really include everything they claim, and may include many things they never mention. How can you find a trusted source of supplements that match their label ingredients with what is in the tablets? To choose a company that you can trust, you need to do your homework and make sure they are following the highest production standards available for supplement manufacturers. Here are a few points to consider:

- Is a scientist the founder?
- Does the company support an international vision of health?
- Does the company focus on prevention, as well as research and development year after year?
- Does the company follow the technological advances and new discoveries?
- Do they clinically test their products for pureness and safety, potency, and bioavailability?
- Does the company use clinical tests to determine absorbability of their products within the body?
- Do they work with a large team of scientists on a full-time basis?
- Does the company control the manufacturing process in their facilities, thus being able to control the quality of the raw ingredients and the finally produced supplements?
- Does the company have certifications from third parties that have global recognition, such as Good Manufacturing Practices (GMP), Therapeutic Goods Administration (TGA), NSF International, Consumer Lab.com, and others? Are these certifications listed on their website or other marketing materials?
- Do they work in partnership with other renowned research centers, universities, and hospitals?
- Do they focus on personalization, recognizing that every person is unique?

As you can see, the company that you choose to provide your supplements needs to demonstrate their efforts to maintain quality through all areas of their process. If they cannot show this type of control, it may not be worth spending your time and money on their product. But let's discuss one vitamin that you access simply by stepping outside.

The Famous SUN VITAMIN : A Source of Vitamin D

Do you know the importance of this particular vitamin? I can tell you that I SEE the difference in my clinic on a seasonal basis. In October and November, when the days are beginning to shorten, my clients are more tired, with mood symptoms, such as depression, and can be less patient, more irritable, and have less tolerance about their pain, and can be easily discouraged. These symptoms seem to disappear with the onset of spring and the return of long sunny days.

How do you react when the sun reappears after a few days of rain? How is your mood? Does your day become more enjoyable because of the sunshine? Do you tend to try to go outside to see the sun more often?

Did you know that the French study, SUVIMAX, showed that, beyond 50 years old, 80% of women showed a deficiency related to reduced vitamin D production capacity within the skin?

When exposed to UVB rays, your skin produces Vitamin D. In northern latitudes, the summer gives us between 10h and 14h of sunshine daily. According to some studies, there is a deficiency in some North Americans even when the sun shines. How is this possible? If you are like most people, especially if you work in an office or if you never leave the house without covering your skin in sunscreen, then your skin is rarely touched by those UVB rays. Did you also know that men and women with dark skin have a higher risk of developing severe vitamin D deficiency? The reason is that the greater amount of pigmentation within the skin inhibits the synthesis of vitamin D, by blocking UVB rays just like a sunscreen[5]. Highly pigmented skin can make vitamin D precursors, but the more pigment there is, the more sun exposure is required. You also should not forget the people who come from other cultures, with clothing that covers them from head to foot, thus not exposing any of their skin to the sun.

Once again, I recommend a supplement of vitamin D. Vitamin D3, instead of D2, should be reflected in the supplement because that is more effective within your system. You also should check to see if the brand has the proper certifications.

Many researchers have studied vitamin D and demonstrated its role in maintaining many aspects of health. These include building up the immune system to fight colds and flus; chronic obstructive pulmonary disease; bone health; cancer; nervous system issues, such as language disorders, cognitive decline, Alzheimer's, multiple sclerosis, depression; diabetes; fibromyalgia; and miscarriages. This list is just a small example that shows the importance of meeting our daily vitamin D requirements. Here are some more areas where vitamin D provides benefits or plays a critical physiological role:

Do you know that vitamin D is also an active steroid hormone that can control genes?

It has been shown to modify the expression of 1,000 different genes in the body, which is roughly 5% of the human protein encoding genome.

Do you know that Vitamin D controls serotonin production? Serotonin, commonly known as the happiness hormone, is a chemical messenger in the central nervous system that is involved in many physiological functions, such as sleep, aggression, eating, and sexual behavior, as well as depression. Therefore, not only is vitamin D important for your physiological well-being, it is also key to your emotional well-being!

Do you know that vitamin D plays a major role in calcium metabolism? Calcium supplements work best in combination with vitamin D, thus maximizing the effects of both supplements.

Do you know the importance of vitamin D with pregnant women? Vitamin D may protect the newborn against the development of type 1 diabetes[6]. Also, vitamin

D provided through the mother may influence the child's language skills[7][8]. Vitamin D also has beneficial effects regarding the bone structure, since it significantly increases bone mineral content for the child[9]. There is also a link between Vitamin D deficiency and autism[10].

These are just a few of the areas where research has shown the benefits of vitamin D. Others may come to light as research continues in this area. However, it is important to note that this is a vitamin that is necessary to provide your body, on a daily basis, to join the health epidemic!

The MULTIVITAMIN is One of the Solutions!

As you can see, there is truly a long list of reasons to supplement to keep your body in optimal health. Your system can suffer from a lack of vital nutrients that are reduced or missing altogether from your food supply. You need many vitamins, minerals, and antioxidants. This list includes A, B1, B2, B3, B5, B6, B8, B9, B12, C, D, E, K, calcium, magnesium, potassium, iodine, zinc, selenium, silicon, copper, manganese, chromium, molybdenum, vanadium, boron, coenzyme Q10, alpha lipoic acid, and many others.

The multivitamin provides a balance to your cells, rounding out their daily needs. Each day, your cells generate new ones and renew older ones. You do need vital nutrients daily; there is no question. Therefore, it's a necessary part of a good daily routine. Multivitamins complete what is lacking on your plate, essentially working in tandem with your plate. The benefits include metabolizing your food even better!

Logically, how can your body work effectively if your cells are missing nutrients? If you could see your cells every day and see the consequences in real time, would you make a change to your lifestyle and eating habits? Probably! You cannot see the effect on your cells. Thus, you lack the motivation to make changes in your lifestyle. We all need a wake-up call!

MY MISSION:

I want to impact your health and to steer you toward true health, an OPTIMAL HEALTH!

To do this, you must learn things that will motivate you to make changes in your lifestyle, making you a part of the health epidemic!

You should compare your body to an assembly line. All products are the result of many steps, and each step is important. Missing or skipping steps can be catastrophic!

You will not end up with the same product if steps are missed or reversed.

It's the same for your mind and body. If you skip steps necessary for optimal health, then you shouldn't ask why you are tired, have digestive problems, pain, and a host of other diseases or problems.

Marginal or subclinical micronutrient deficiencies have been linked to general fatigue,[11] impaired immunity[12] [13], and adverse effects on cognition[14]. There are myriads of campaigns on nutrition that try to convince to make better food choices. The reality is that most Americans eat an energy-rich, nutrient-poor diet with a lack of fruits and vegetables[15]. Micronutrients deficiencies are widespread in the U.S., Canada, and around the world. Our bad habits are difficult to change, and most people lack the knowledge and motivation to facilitate that change.

Do not think that multivitamins are made equal. Many contain synthetic micronutrients, which may not be absorbed, do not work in synergy with the body, and may contain contaminants, heavy metals, petroleum products, pesticides, and sugar. With these types of ingredients, they are often more harmful than beneficial to your health! Using them is the same as throwing your money down the drain.

When you choose a multivitamin, it must contain a large spectrum of minerals, trace elements, vitamins, and antioxidants. This multivitamin should be complete, with high quality, highly bioavailable, effective, balanced, and optimal dosages of nutrients. It should also offer a guarantee of purity. Many people think that they can just mix all nutrients without any research or study, and produce a multivitamin that can be effective. Science, however, proves this wrong. High quality ingredients and balanced micronutrients are needed.

I consume a multivitamin of the highest quality, two times a day. The reason is that some vitamins are water soluble, such as vitamins B and C, so they are excreted out of the body rapidly. It's better to repeat the process with a second dose to make sure all the cells are getting what they need.

Here are a few things to keep in mind when choosing a multivitamin, regarding the nutrients offered:

- Check that the supplement contains the natural form of vitamin E: D-alpha-tocopherol versus the synthetic isomeric form: D-L-alpha tocopherol.
- Don't take a multivitamin that contains iron because if you don't have an iron deficiency, it could be dangerous for your health. Have a blood test to determine if your iron is low and needs to be supplemented. If you do have a deficiency, your doctor can prescribe a dose of iron to fit your circumstances.
- Another vitamin that you must be cautious with is VITAMIN A. At its highest level, there is a risk of toxicity and accumulation. The better choice is to take a multivitamin with a mix of beta-carotene and vitamin A. Beta-carotene is a precursor of vitamin A, designated provitamin A.

- Choose chelated minerals, because they are easier to digest and are best in organic forms, such as gluconate, citrate, picolinate, and fumarate.
- You also need a variety of antioxidants and phytonutrients. These are scientifically proven to protect your cells against oxidative stress, which is one of the key reasons that often leads to diseases. Bioflavonoids, coenzyme Q10, turmeric, lipoic acid alpha, lycopene, green tea extract, zeaxanthin, and lutein are all better if they are standardized extracts.

As you can see, it's not so simple to find the best multivitamin to insure your optimal health. It is possible if you do your homework. As previously mentioned, supplements need to be made with high quality ingredients in the right doses to have the best effects. Now that I have explored why food cannot be our only source of nutrition, and some facts to be aware of regarding supplements, it's time to explore nutrition and how our bodies process the nutrients and toxins that we expose ourselves to daily.

---

[1] PRE-POLLUTED : A report on the toxic substances in the umbilical cord blood of Canadian newborns.
[2] Canadian Cancer Society's Advisory Committee on Cancer Statistics. Canadian Cancer Statistics 2015. Toronto, ON: Canadian Cancer Society; 2015.
[3] Hathcock JN, Azzi A, Blumberg J, Bray T, Dickinson A, Frei B, Jialal I, Johnston CS, Kelly FJ, Kraemer K, Packer L, Parthasarathy S, Sies H, Traber MG. Vitamins E and C are safe across a broad range of intakes. American Journal of Clinical Nutrition. 2005 Apr;81(4):736-45. Review. PubMed PMID: 15817846.

[4] Micallef MA, Munro IA, Garg ML. An inverse relationship between plasma n-3 fatty acids and C-reactive protein in healthy individuals. Eur J Clin Nutr. 2009 Sep;63(9):1154-6. Epub 2009 Apr 8. PubMed PMID: 19352379.

[5] Laura M. Hall, Michael G. Kimlin, Pavel A. Aronov, Bruce D. Hammock, James R. Slusser, Leslie R. Woodhouse, and Charles B. Stephensen. Vitamin D Intake Needed to Maintain Target Serum 25-Hydroxyvitamin D Concentrations in Participants with Low Sun Exposure and Dark Skin Pigmentation Is Substantially Higher Than Current Recommendations. Journal of Nutrition, first published on Jan 6, 2010 as doi: doi:10.3945/jn.109.115253.

[6] Sørensen IM, Joner G, Jenum PA, Eskild A, Torjesen PA, Stene LC. Maternal serum levels of 25-hydroxy-vitamin D, during pregnancy and risk of type 1 diabetes in the offspring. Diabetes. 2012 Jan;61(1):175-8. Epub 2011 Nov 28. PubMed PMID: 22124461; PubMed Central PMCID: PMC3237654.

[7] Kids' Language Skills Tied to Mom's Vitamin D. By Todd Neale, Senior Staff Writer, MedPage Today, February 13, 2012.

[8] Whitehouse AJ, Holt BJ, Serralha M, Holt PG, Kusel MM, Hart PH. Maternal serum vitamin D levels during pregnancy and offspring neurocognitive development. Pediatrics. 2012 Mar;129(3):485-93. Epub 2012 Feb 13. PubMed PMID: 22331333.

[9] Javaid MK, Crozier SR, Harvey NC, et al. Maternal vitamin D status during pregnancy and childhood bone mass at age 9 years: a longitudinal study. Lancet 2006; 367(9504): 36–43.

[10] Report: Vitamin D Regulates Serotonin: Role in Autism by Rhonda Perciavalle Patrick, Ph.D.

[11] Huskisson E, Maggini S, Ruf M. The role of vitamins and minerals in energy metabolism and well-being. J Int Med Res. 2007;35(3):277-289. (PubMed)

[12] Ibs K-H, Rink L. Zinc. In: Hughes DA, Darlington LG, Bendich A,eds. Diet and human immune function. Totowa: Human Press Inc.; 2004:241-259.

[13] Bhaskaram P. Immunobiology of mild micronutrient deficiencies. Br J Nutr. 2001;85 Suppl 2:S75-80. (PubMed)

[14] Eussen SJ, de Groot LC, Joosten LW, et al. Effect of oral vitamin B-12 with or without folic acid on cognitive function in older people with mild vitamin B-12 deficiency: a randomized, placebo-controlled trial. Am J Clin Nutr. 2006;84(2):361-370. (PubMed)

[15] Centers for Disease Control and Prevention. State indicator report on fruits and vegetables, 2009.

http://www.fruitsandveggiesmatter.gov/indicatorreport. Accessed 8/23/11.

Chapter 2

NUTRITION

The Long Route of Your Digestive System

A s a human being, you know how important your digestive system is and how quickly it works. All the individual organs have their tasks but also work together in harmony to make up your entire digestive system.

When I speak at a conference, I like to ask attendees this question: where do you think that digestion begins? Most people will say the mouth. While that is true in part, it primarily begins in your brain first (specifically your hypothalamus). When you see a succulent and gorgeous chocolate cake, the hypothalamus in your brain will stimulate your appetite, thus causing your mouth to produce saliva.

The main organs involved in digestion are your mouth, stomach, liver, gallbladder, pancreas, small intestine, and colon. If you want to optimize your health, you really must take care of your digestive system. It's the key! All your organs work together to convert food into energy and basic nutrients that feed your entire body. Don't forget that your organs are also a group of cells, which are nourished from the digestive system. Your organs also need nourishment. It's logical! Your incredible digestive system also includes nerves, hormones, bacteria, and blood, yet everything must work in synergy. Here's an example of how it all works together to nourish our bodies.

When you see a delicious chocolate cake, your brain sends signals to your mouth, so you start salivating. The saliva in your mouth mixes with food and begins to break it down to a form that is more easily absorbed, known as the food bowl. When you swallow, your food bowl is pushed into the esophagus and goes down to the stomach. In your mouth, it's important to break down the food into easily digested pieces. In your saliva, you also have enzymes that help to break down your food as you chew. You must chew something 30 to 40 times for each bit to be mixed well with the enzymes. It's one of the keys involved in your digestion.

The next organ is your stomach, which is a storage tank for food. Your stomach transforms the food bowl into chyme by using gastric juices, which contain digestive enzymes, hydrochloric acid (HCL), and mucus. Your stomach is like a mixer and grinder during this process.

But keep in mind that your stomach does not have teeth! Therefore, you need to chew well to maximize the digestion of your food during this process. Consider chewing your food at least 30 times. This process makes it easier for your stomach to do its job. Eventually, the semi-fluid mass or chyme is sent to your small intestine. If your stomach isn't doing the job right, your small intestine will have to work even harder.

What could be contributing to your stomach not doing its job? It could be stomach issues due to missing digestive enzymes, and/or you may not have enough HCL.

Now, let's discuss another critical part of the digestive system, which is the liver. It is the second largest organ in your body. Its primary function is to produce the bile released into your small intestine. This bile emulsifies fats, transforming fat into fat droplets. Your liver will also cleanse and purify your blood. In fact, all the blood in your body passes through the liver. As a result, everything that you eat, breathe, and put on your skin will eventually end up passing through your liver.

This organ breaks down and stores amino acids, as well as synthesizing and metabolizing fats and cholesterol, plus storing glucose. Your liver can also store iron and B12. If you have a deficiency in this mineral and this vitamin, check your liver function.

After you absorb approximately 90% of the nutrients in your small intestines, those nutrients enter your bloodstream and are sent to your liver for filtering and detoxification. If you want to support your liver, eat organic foods and avoid the toxic ones. Be careful, especially with meat and dairy products, because of the amount of antibiotics, growth hormones, steroids, and other chemicals stored in the meat due to the diet of the cows and other animals.

Fermented foods also support the liver and gall bladder, such as apple cider vinegar, kefir, sauerkraut, kimchi, goat's milk, and goat's yogurt. Turmeric is also beneficial in detoxifying the liver. So many benefits are available with this extraordinary spice. We can't forget the herb, milk thistle. According to University of Maryland Medical Center, several scientific studies suggest that substances in milk thistle (especially a flavonoid called silymarin) protect the liver from toxins, including certain drugs, such as acetaminophen (Tylenol) that if taken in high doses can cause liver damage. Silymarin also has antioxidant and anti-inflammatory properties. Also, it may help the liver to repair itself by growing new cells.

The partner organ of your liver is your gall bladder. It's a very small, pear-shaped organ that is used to store and recycle excess bile from your liver. The gallbladder stores bile between meals and plays a key role in the breakdown of fat. See your liver and gallbladder as essentially one symbiotic organ. Many people have their gallbladder removed, and the result is a larger issue regarding their ability to digest and process fats. As a result, you may also need lipase, the enzyme that breaks down fat. It could be a good idea to take digestive enzymes that contains lipase, especially if you have had your gallbladder removed.

If you have liver and gall bladder issues, you should take certain fats like coconut oil, because your body must work less to digest this kind of fat than it does with other fats. I will explain its many benefits later.

Your pancreas is also very important to the digestive process. It secretes digestive enzymes (lipase, amylase, protease, etc) and bicarbonates ions that it pours into your duodenum. It also secretes hormones, such as insulin and glucagon, which are essential for controlling the amount of sugar in your blood.

If you have a blood sugar issue, such as diabetes, it typically indicates there is a problem in the pancreas. Your pancreas plays a role in creating and producing enzymes and hormones, which are necessary for your body and systems to function properly.

Your pancreatic juice joins the common duct, which allows bile to help break down fat before it reaches your small intestine. If your body isn't producing enough enzymes, it will affect the breakdown of all your food (carbohydrates, fats, and proteins).

Every step in your digestive tract is important, but there is one that is more important than all the others.

Your Second Brain

Have you ever heard about the second brain? This second brain is your intestines because such a large portion of your nervous system is located here. Your digestive system interacts with other systems within your body in a similar fashion to your nervous system and endocrine system, which is so important for hormone balance. There is also a tie to your immune system. Do you know that 70–80% of your immune system relies on your gut?

Your small intestine is crucial to the digestive process. This 20-foot-long passageway moves food from the acidic environment of the stomach to the more alkaline environment of the small intestine. You have protrusions, or villi, for increasing the overall surface area, which helps to keep food moving toward your colon. You have enzymes on your villi that assist in the further breakdown of nutrients into a readily absorbable form. It also helps to prevent leaky gut, a discovery and a new term used to explain damage to the bowel lining or small intestine lining.

It can happen if your organs aren't functioning well due to a poor and inflammatory diet, fungal infections, parasite infections, toxins in your system, medications, and undigested food, and the list could go on.

According to research published in the International Journal of Gastroenterology and Hepatology 2006, intestinal permeability (leaky gut) has been linked to autoimmune diseases, including type 1 diabetes, Crohn's disease, and dermatitis.

All the folds in the small intestines are meant to maximize the digestion of food and nutrient absorption. Each part of the small intestine plays a critical role in the digestive process.

The leftovers from the small intestine travel to your colon or large intestine, which is about 5 feet long. Although 90 % of the nutrient absorption occurs inside the small intestine, a lot of fat and soluble vitamins, as well as some minerals, can also be absorbed in the colon. You also have gut bacteria, called flora or probiotics, which continue to help the digestion. They're really important for detoxifying.

Your stool is formed by food debris, toxins, bacteria, and fibers. You need plenty of colon probiotics and healthy fats. As I discussed in the last chapter, probiotics nourish your colon.

NEW DISCOVERY : Your Microbioma

Did you hear about the microbioma? It's a new discovery. Research has found that we are made of bacteria and cells. Some scientists talk about a ratio of up to 10:1; there can be ten times more bacteria than cells. Of course, all these researchers are not in agreement. For the moment, the only thing that we can say is that the two worlds work together.

Have you heard about the fecal transplant? It involves transferring stool from a healthy person to the intestine of an unhealthy or sick person. It is similar to an organ transplant. They have found that a microbiota that lives in the intestines is similar to an organ. There are studies on this topic, and it could completely change the life of a person.

It's a symbiotic relationship between the probiotics in your colon and you. Your probiotics help you to break down and digest your food, producing B12, butyrate, and vitamin K2, creating enzymes that destroy harmful bacteria, crowding out bad bacteria, yeast, and fungi, and stimulating secretion of IgA and regulatory T-cells.

A study from Stanford School of Medicine (Stanford University Medical Center) found that consuming probiotics can increase vitamin B12 levels, as much as 67%! Source: http://sm.stanford.edu/archive/stanmed/2009fall/upfront.html

The majority of the probiotics in your body are all located in your colon. Do you understand now why it is so crucial to take care of the colon by taking probiotics?

Taking an excellent quality probiotic supplement can be one of the better choices to take care of your microbiota. It's also a good idea to include plenty of fibers from multiple sources, including psyllium and inulin. It's important because different types of fiber provide specific benefits. The occidental diet is missing key fibers. Fibers, called prebiotics, also feed probiotics.

Again, if you take prebiotics and probiotics by supplement, take care in choosing the source. There are too many that contain contaminants, which are mixed with other substances while not providing a complete variety.

You Are What You Digest

You are what you eat. Is it true? If it's true, then why do two people who eat the same things have different reactions? For one person, it could give him energy, vitality, and plenty of benefits, but for the other person, no increased energy, no vitality, headaches, and even some digestive issues. The question is, why?

The reason is because YOU ARE WHAT YOU DIGEST!

If you followed what I have explained previously, the digestive system is a very crucial, long road. If the second person doesn't assimilate the food correctly, the result will be different for that person. Now you understand why it is so important to have a healthy digestive system!!!

If you eat crap, you will feel like garbage, you will look like garbage, and you will smell like garbage. Why? Simply put, it is because you will be digesting garbage. Where are you getting your nutrients? If you decide to exchange your bad habits for good habits, you will become a person who eats very well. Unfortunately, you cannot just change your habits. You also need to clean out the garbage from your system due to your past bad habits, using a detox.

The DETOX is a Must!

The word, *detox*, is popular in our world. With all the toxic food, processed food, pesticides, antibiotics, medication, toxins, bad fats, sugar, and so much more, it's difficult to have optimal health. I see so many digestive issues, such as constipation and congested livers, in my office. Clearing out the garbage is critical to improving your digestive health in the short and long term.

Why Should You Consider a Detox?

- Digestive problems
- Allergies
- Decreased energy
- Obesity or overweight
- Skin problems
- Eliminating toxins
- Cleaning the organs (liver, kidneys, skin, small intestines, colon)

What are the benefits of a detox?

- Cleans out the liver by helping to filter and eliminate toxins
- Improves vitality and energy
- Improves circulation
- Improves overall health
- Improves digestion, assimilation, and elimination

When should you do a detox?

- NOW if you have never done a detox before, or it has been a long time
- SPRING (when the liver is at its maximum energy according to Chinese medicine, so the detoxification occurs in more depth)
- FALL (in preparation for the winter)
- January (after your holidays because you ate fatter and sweeter foods, as well as consuming more alcohol)
- DISEASE or ANESTHESIA (substances stay in the blood for at least six months)
- AFTER THE HOLIDAYS (because you need to let go of the bad eating habits of the holidays!)

Keep in mind that once you do a detox, it is important to make changes to your habits to limit the garbage reentering your system. Next, I am going to share with you the 5R program for detox, which supports you in making changes to optimize your health.

The Program 5R for Detoxing

1) REMOVE the toxins. It includes the bad food and drink choices, environmental toxins, bacteria, parasites, yeasts and chemical agents in your personal and household products and your foods. I like to use milk thistle, N-Acetyl L-Cystein, alpha lipoic acid, green tea, and turmeric for extra help. A good book to read about this topic is THE HEALTHY HOME.

2) REPLACE bad foods with whole foods that have plenty enzymes and fibers. I like to use a complete complex of digestive enzymes, as well as soluble and insoluble fibers. Also FILL IN deficiencies such as a lack of hydrochloric acid, vitamin D, zinc, pancreatic enzymes, magnesium, omega 3 and other missing nutrients. These nutrients allow the body to work well.

3) REINOCULATE and RESEED with good bacteria to help your digestive flora and immune system. At this step, you need probiotics, fermented foods, germination, fibers, and prebiotics.

4) REPAIR with amino acid L-glutamine, which helps repair the intestinal lining. It allows a faster multiplication. Homemade chicken bone and beef broths are also great in repairing the gut lining (mucous).

5) REBALANCING AND MAINTAINING your new lifestyle. You must consider each of the following aspects:

- Healthy nutrition
- Supplementation (to fill the gaps)
- Deep sleep (Make sure you sleep well because your body does a lot of repairs at night.)
- Stress management
- Regular physical activity
- Positive thinking

For additional help, I like to use various supplements because we live in a toxic world. During a detox, it's even more important that you choose supplements with a guarantee of purity and efficency! Many don't work because they contain contaminants and other things that you don't want, and they defeat the purpose of the detox.

Join the movement on sparknflynow.com to know more about DETOX.

Coconut Oil Everywhere!

Not all saturated fat is bad for you. Plant-based saturated fats, such as those found in coconut oil, provide some health benefits. COCONUT OIL is one of the fats that contains the most medium-chain triglycerides (MCTs). Due to their shorter chain length, MCTs can be absorbed easily in the gastrointestinal tract and transported directly to the liver to produce energy.

Coconut oil is more readily digested, absorbed, and metabolized than either animal fats or vegetable oils, which primarily contain long-chain triglycerides. It could be an excellent source of fat, especially for individuals with fat malabsorption disorders. Unlike the other types of fat, pancreatic enzymes and bile are not even necessary for the digestion of medium-chain triglycerides (MCTs) inside the coconut oil.

According to Bruce Fife, N.D., "Coconut oil is the healthiest oil on earth."

"Coconut oil is the healthiest oil you can use," said Joseph Mercola, D.O.

These are just two experts who support the use of coconut oil. You can see a variety of studies on the topic at www.coconutresearchcenter.org. Here are some of the benefits of Coconut Oil:

- Antimicrobial Effects
- Cancer
- Cardiovascular Health
- Diabetes
- Digestion and Nutrient Absorption
- Epilepsy, Alzheimer's, and other Neurological Disorders
- HIV/AIDS, and Sexually Transmitted Diseases
- Hospital Patient Care/Enteral and Parenteral Nutrition
- Intestinal Health
- Kidney Health
- Liver Health
- Malabsorption Syndromes
- Metabolism/Energy
- Skin Health
- Weight Management

Since MCTs have less of an opportunity for deposition into adipose tissue, they have been used successfully to support healthy weight management programs.

You can use coconut oil almost everywhere. It has the advantage of not producing toxic compounds when heated. Therefore, it is a preferred oil for cooking. Choose coconut oil instead of the other oils to cook. You can use it as a replacement for butter, other oils, and milk, as well as on your toast, to cook your eggs, and in your smoothies, coffees, teas, and desserts, or simply take it naturally.

If you train or are an athlete who likes to make smoothies, or you are searching for high quality protein, fat, and carbohydrate-based shakes, choose those that contain lipids in the form of coconut oil. As I've mentioned before, medium-chain triglycerides (MCTs) do not require bile and pancreatic enzymes to be digested! Therefore, your body can concentrate on everything else, improving your body's performance. Your liver converts coconut oil into ENERGY. It provides a clear advantage for you, especially if you want to be productive, effective, and performant.

The Glycemic Index : The New Trend for Controlling Your Weight and Your Health

You have probably heard about the glycemic index before. Do you know that this is a key to truly maintaining an ideal healthy weight and also overall health? Maybe you're one of those people who have at some time in your life tried all sorts of diets, without success, or rather with limited success. Maybe you have played yoyo with your weight for a big part of your life.

The secret to losing weight is no longer in calorie counting. We must now look at the glycemic index of foods. Stop limiting yourself by thinking in terms of CALORIES. So many diets teach this today. What really matters is the GLYCEMIC INDEX of your food! If you make the right choices, you will be satisfied and healthier. The term, *blood sugar*, refers to the measurement of glucose in your blood. The glycemic index is a way to rank foods based on the rate at which your blood sugar rises in your blood following ingestion of that food.

The more the glycemic index of a food is high, the faster your sugar count will rise in your blood.

Imagine you eat high-glycemic foods, such as a bran muffin or a slice of white or brown bread, each of which you think are healthy. The sugar in your blood will quickly rise until you reach what is called the glycemic peak. At this moment, your brain sends a message to your pancreas to secrete large amounts of insulin. It's a hormone that participates very actively in the storage of glucose in the liver and the muscles in the form of glycogen. This glycogen is therefore a reserve. However, the extra sugar will be stored as fat in your fat cells (adipocytes).

You will find yourself with a very low level of sugar in your blood. Thus, you may experience a state of discomfort, fatigue, difficulty concentrating, headache, impulsiveness, sugar rage, mood changes, and even aggressivity. If you are hungry, you might not worry about choosing wisely, but instead, eat the first thing that falls into your hands, even if it is a high glycemic index food. But this just keeps the cycle going. In the long term, your pancreas still works very hard to reduce your blood sugar. Additionally, many will end up with an accumulation of fat around the abdomen, buttocks, and hips as a result. If you want to have energy, stay with mostly low-glycemic foods.

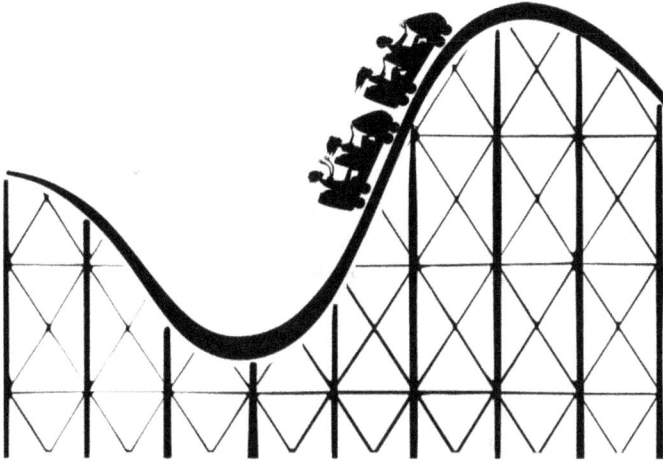

THE ROLLER COASTER

There is a danger in repeatedly making extreme ups and downs with your blood sugar. It's like doing the famous roller coaster with your blood sugar.

With time, you may become resistant to your own insulin. At the slightest intake of sugar, your pancreas works all the time; it never has a rest! So, you end up with extra pounds, and you have an increased difficulty losing weight.

Also, the body creates inflammation; then comes the metabolic syndrome, diabetes, and degenerative diseases.

Choosing to eat low-glycemic foods provides many advantages. It allows you to maintain your ideal weight, feel a satiety that lasts longer, eat your fill, and maintain a good energy level (and no longer feel the crash), as well as reducing inflammatory reactions in your body, and ending, once and for all, calorie counting.

Studies have shown that people who begin the morning with a high-glycemic index breakfast consume more calories throughout their day, versus those who eat a low-glycemic index breakfast.

Make it a habit to choose low-glycemic foods (G.I) under 55. You can find a multitude of pictures on the web giving you the glycemic index of various foods.

For example, you can start your day with an omelet with vegetables and half an avocado. Another interesting alternative is to consume a good smoothie or shake in the morning! Water or homemade almond milk, some frozen organic fruits, and superfoods, such as goji berry and spirulina, plus based plant protein, like protein from peas and potatoes, are a great start to your day. Make sure that your plant-based protein does not contain artificial flavors, artificial sweeteners, artificial colors, contaminants, and toxins. They must follow GMP standards. Make sure it is low glycemic and that they offer a guarantee of purity, to be truly beneficial. The one I'm taking is made with raw ingredients, using the highest manufacturing quality, the highest purity and potency, and has third party validation.

The Harvard Pyramid Tells You

For Canadians, you know the famous Canadian food guide! For Americans, you also have your guide! In fact, many countries have their own food guide. Are they really guides that can help you maintain good health or improve your health?

I prefer the healthy eating pyramid, published by faculty members at the Harvard School of Public Health.

It has been developed according to the latest research on nutrition, giving you a resource to help fuel your body effectively.

For more information about The Healthy Eating Plate, please see The Nutrition Source, Department of Nutrition, Harvard School of Public Health, www.thenutrition source.org, and Harvard Health Publications, www.health .harvard.edu.

I appreciate this pyramid a lot. At its basis, the emphasis is on aspects such as lifestyle health, daily exercise, and weight control.

You can see the importance of:

Vegetables and fruits, healthy fats and oil, whole grains, nuts and seeds, beans, tofu, fish, poultry, and eggs. *Be careful with soy because you have to choose soy without GMO.

Researchers place much less emphasis on dairy products, red meats, and other products. These products must be limited because they have been associated with different health issues. Science talks. There are other solutions.

You can see red wine is also for those who drink (but be careful because it's in moderation and not for everyone).

You can see that they also put MULTIVITAMIN with an EXTRA VITAMIN D SUPPLEMENT as a recommendation for most of the people. Why? Because of the research, which demonstrates that we really need it!

The only thing I want to add again: be careful of the quality of the multivitamin. See Chapter 1 to choose the best one for you.

I love this pyramid, and I sincerely think that it is the healthiest option of all the guides available. Joining the *epidemic of healthy people* starts with changing your food choices and what you are putting into your body. Making the right choices, which include organic options and avoiding processed foods, can make a huge difference in how your body functions and how you feel!

Chapter 3

INFLAMMATION EATS YOU

Inflammation - Your Silent Killer!

As an osteopath and former physiotherapist, I treat and have treated many people with musculoskeletal and orthopedic conditions. I am very familiar with the concept of inflammation. Perhaps you are one of those people who believe that inflammation can only be detected by these following signs: redness, pain, swelling, heat. Yes, these are significant clinical signs that confirm inflammation. However, this is not always the case.

Inflammation is a natural defense from your body against pathogens and injuries, so it is an extremely important process. It is normal when it is temporary. However, when inflammation persists and becomes chronic, it could cause serious damage.

Let's return to the 4 clinical signs. Do you see those signs when you are diagnosed with cancer? Not at all! You do not necessarily have redness, pain, swelling, and heat to signal that something is wrong before cancer is diagnosed. This is called silent inflammation. This inflammation eats your insides like rust does on a car. The consequences of this type of inflammation can be disastrous!

Silent inflammation is a chronic process that allows your body to turn against itself. Your immune system attacks you. Your little soldiers, which are supposed to protect you, turn against you and attack your organs and cells. Inflammation starts destroying your tissues.

Imagine an ember in a fire that is constantly being fed, or an open wound that does not heal because it is constantly being irritated. Your arteries, your diverse cells, your nerve cells, your organs, and so on, are all damaged by the embers; and, eventually, it compromises your immune system. The damage that ensues can eventually turn into degenerative diseases, including cancer.

Inflammation is often the cause of a variety of diseases, such as cancer, cardiovascular disease, Alzheimer's, type 2 diabetes, arthritis, autoimmune diseases, neurological diseases, lung diseases, and so on.

You can't imagine the huge impact that you can have on inflammation by changing your nutritional intake and consuming supplements of the best quality!

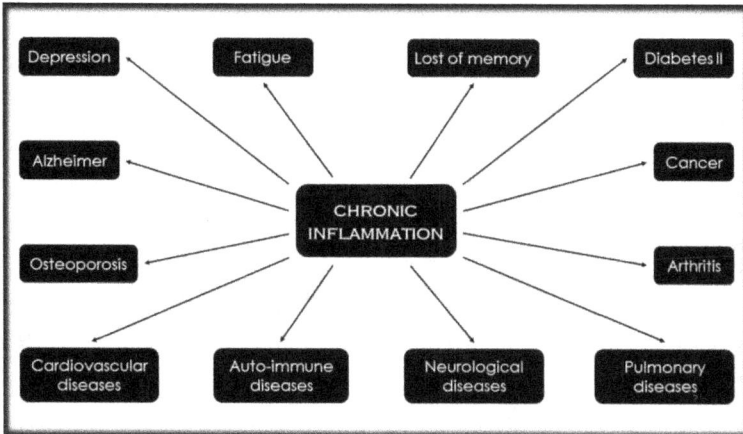

But what are the real causes of this inflammation that is so destructive?

There are several. You remember in the introduction when I mentioned that our environment is no longer the same today. Instead, it is full of contaminants: pesticides and herbicides found in our food; chemical agents that we find in the water, land, and air; heavy metals, such as mercury, lead, and arsenic; and pollution. All of these factors contribute to this silent inflammation.

What about the processed food that is so prevalent in our culture? Today, most of the food is distinctly acidic, such as dairy products, red meat, and sugar. These are three categories of highly acidifying foods for your body, which can cause significant damage over time to your body.

If you are like most people, vegetables (especially greens that are very alkaline) and fruits have no special place in your daily life. Yet they have to be a big part in protecting your body and helping it to achieve the right balance.

That's not all…

Did you also know that an imbalance of essential fatty acids can truly destroy your tissues? They are called eicosanoids, which are derived from two essential fatty acids, linoleic acid and alpha-linolenic acid. They play a vital role in regulating the level of inflammation in your body, as some are inflammatory, and others are anti-inflammatory. An imbalance causes systemic inflammation.

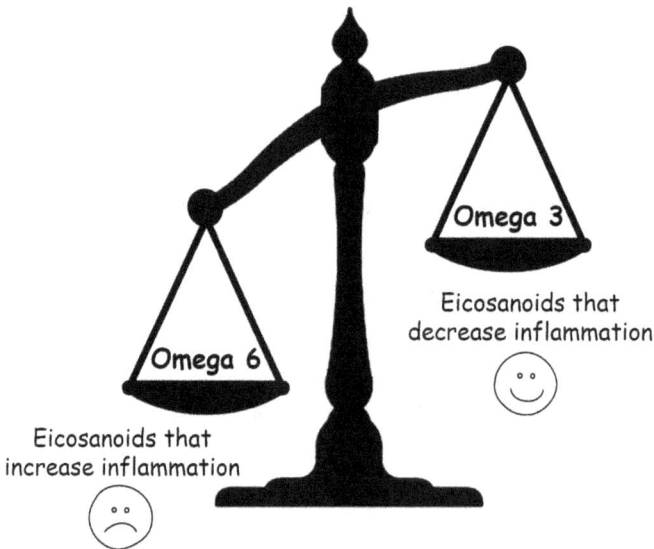

Omega 3
Eicosanoids that decrease inflammation

Omega 6
Eicosanoids that increase inflammation

Imagine a scale with 2 sides. On one side, there are the inflammatory eicosanoids, and on the other side, anti-inflammatory eicosanoids. There must always be a balance between stimulating and mitigating the inflammatory response.

Omega-6 is a type of eicosanoid, which increases inflammation, while omega 3 is a type of eicosanoid that decreases inflammation. If your intake of omega 6 is higher than your omega 3, you will produce more inflammation. As I mentioned to you in Chapter 1, today's Western diet is a clear imbalance between omega 6 and omega 3. The report omega 6/ omega 3 ratio should be around 1 for 1. Today, it is not surprising to find ratios up to 20, 30, and even 40 for 1. Catastrophic for your organism!

You must therefore increase your intake of omega 3. Fish is an excellent source of omega 3, but what about the heavy metals it contains? We should consume it in moderation (about 2-3 times per week), and focus on smaller fish that contain less heavy metals. What can we do on the other days to protect ourselves from this inflammation?

As I mentioned before, I recommend taking daily supplements of omega 3 from marine sources to provide you with what you need to combat this destructive inflammation. Their virtues are too important to do without them.

Do not forget the importance of consuming omega 3 CERTIFIED TO HAVE NO HEAVY METALS. You will be surprised that most companies do not have this certification. The process is very expensive, which makes it harder to obtain. But to obtain the best product, you need to make sure that you have it.

If you are not convinced that inflammation is a killer, look at *Time Magazine*, from February 23, 2004!

Gluten – Is it Really a Fad?

Maybe you are fed up with hearing about gluten, or you think that it's just a fad. My goal here is just that you become aware of certain realities in regard to this topic.

First, you must know exactly what gluten is. I am often amused by the responses of people who think they know what gluten is but who seem to be very misinformed.

GLUTEN is simply the protein contained in the grains of many cereals, such as wheat, barley, rye, kamut, and spelt. By its structure, gluten gives an elastic consistency to the dough that is made with flour from these grains. This is why many give it the abbreviation, GLUE (meaning glue). Gluten consists of two families of proteins: prolamins and glutelins. Prolamin of wheat is called gliadin.

It is a pity that it is not possible to regain our wild wheat from 10,000 years ago! This former wheat was called Einkorn, and it consisted of 14 chromosomes. With hybridization, wheat proteins have undergone a considerable change of structure. Modern wheat now carries 42 chromosomes. Wheat genetics has changed, and that may be a factor in why we now find so much mild to severe sensitivity and intolerance towards wheat!

Our digestive system has to work much harder than before to digest this protein than it did before.

Another fact to add is mercury intake. Many of you know how mercury can be toxic and destructive to your cells. Mercury is found in fish, seafood, and many other foods, but also in your amalgam fillings. Do you have gray amalgam fillings in your mouth? If that's the case, I highly recommend you have them removed by a holistic dentist (not your conventional dentist who does not care about the fumes and debris that are being released in your mouth).

I invite you to read a valuable book that could transform your life: *A Mouth Full of Poison*, written by Dr. Wentz, a microbiologist. You will find hidden truths about dental amalgam fillings with mercury. My dental profession perspective has changed dramatically, and now I consult a holistic dentist each year. Every time you brush your teeth, eat, or chew gum, mercury particles from these amalgam fillings are escaping into your system. The damage caused by mercury can really affect your health and even bring disease. According to Sanoviv Medical

Institute, if you are already suffering from any disease, the chances of having an effective cure are lower if your mercury level is high.

As you know, mercury is actually toxic. According to Sanoviv Medical Institute, mercury may also result in an inactivation of the enzyme necessary for digestion of gluten. Yet how many people suffer from issues digesting gluten? Perhaps they should be checking their mercury levels, or their exposure to mercury in any form, as part of their gluten intolerance and sensitivity discussion with their doctor.

Keep in mind that Mercury is considered by WHO (World Health Organization) as one of the top ten chemicals or groups of chemicals of major public health concern!

But the gluten of today's wheat may also be causing problems, outside of any issues with mercury. American cardiologist, Dr. William Davis, found that when he removed wheat from his patients' diets, their sugar levels fell consistently, and they lost weight. The chronic asthma, arthritis, and even migraines, depression, lack of energy, inflammation of the digestive system, and skin irritation disappeared. All the patients had a positive change in their health as a result. According to Dr. Davis, gliadin acts on the brain and increases the attention problems, hyperactivity, and concentration issues, as well as mood swings, depression, bipolar disorder, and even schizophrenia.

According to Sanoviv Medical Institute, and several institutes of holistic medicine, GLUTEN may be the source of many diseases and health problems, including:

- Celiac Disease
- Digestive Disorders
- Multiple Sclerosis
- Arthritic Syndromes
- Crohn's Disease
- Ulcerative Colitis
- Celiac Hepatitis
- Diabetes
- Disorders of Thyroid Gland
- Osteoporosis
- Irritable Bowel Syndrome
- Depression/Mood Disorders
- Memory Loss
- Obesity or Weight Gain
- Fibromyalgia
- Skin Disorders
- Schizophrenia
- Headache, Migraine
- Autism
- Attention Disorders With or Without Hyperactivity
- Etc.

More and more people are having a negative response to the gluten. Various symptoms of any kind can be caused by gluten. Do you have trouble digesting or absorbing certain nutrients? Do you suffer from bloating or abdominal pain, diarrhea and/or constipation, flatulence, and nausea with or without vomiting? Do you suffer from fatigue, loss of energy, joint pain, muscle cramps, mouth ulcers, and gastric reflux?

As you can see, symptoms of any kind can be created by this altered gluten. Do not just be satisfied with the test for celiac disease, which is an autoimmune disease induced by gluten ingestion that causes atrophy and destruction of villi in the intestines. In this case, it is an allergy or severe intolerance that can be fatal if you do not avoid gluten.

Know that there is also the gluten sensitivity that you need to consider. It can be mild to severe. If you have the symptoms mentioned above, I strongly recommend you take a more advanced test to assess any gluten sensitivity. You can also do a test by yourself by ceasing gluten for a period of at least one month. If your symptoms abate, then you may have a gluten sensitivity that can be handled best by avoiding gluten altogether. Then, try again by using gluten and seeing if your gluten sensitivity increases.

Remember, today's wheat has been changed at the structural level.

Our flours are processed and then enhanced because the processing does remove the nutrients, and then they must be put back.

I have seen many testimonies of people who have improved their health simply by cutting gluten. What about gluten-free food that is found at the supermarket? Are they any good? NOT AT ALL!

The food industry is fully aware of the need for gluten-free foods, for the reasons I mentioned above. Do you think they benefit? Of course, by creating gluten-free cookies, gluten-free crackers, gluten-free bread, gluten-free dough, gluten-free sauce, gluten-free pastries, gluten-free pasta, gluten-free condiments, and the list goes on. Most are processed foods that have added sugar, artificial sweeteners, artificial colors, artificial flavors, preservatives, and more.

Be aware because gluten-free products often replace the wheat with other types of grains (like corn, soy), which can cause yet another problem with GMOs and altered structures.

The best way to deal with this is to start cooking for yourself. Make your gluten-free bread, pasta, pizza, and desserts. There are so many simple recipes, and your digestive system will be HAPPY and give you more energy as a result.

Are Dairy Products as Good as They Say?

Cow's milk at first seems harmless. Since our childhood, we have drunk it as part of a daily routine; this milk of such whiteness that we were left with a nice little white mustache. According to Robert Cohen, who wrote the book, *Milk – the Deadly Poison*, cow's milk is not quite adapted to the human digestive system. Did you know that cow's milk elevates blood cholesterol and blood fats by its content in cholesterol and polyunsaturated fat?

According to Cohen, dairy products that older people would absorb are one of the main causes of osteoporosis. Pasteurization and uperisation make a denatured product and biocidique (food destructive of life). Milk contains 300 times more casein (cow's milk protein) than breast milk. Do you think that's normal?

Many researchers believe that casein is the main substance responsible for joint inflammation that is seen in rheumatoid arthritis. It is the reason why the abolition of milk products can improve the condition of people suffering from this type of arthritis.

The multinational Monsanto produces a hormone designed to increase milk production. Thus, milk production increased from 10 liters a day to almost 50 liters in the USA. Unfortunately, this also leads the cows to have more infections, thus increasing the use of antibiotics in these animals.

According to Cohen, the antibiotic levels are 100 times higher than a few years ago. In the USA, nearly 50% of antibiotics are reserved for cattle. If these poor cows consume these hormones and antibiotics, then you eat cheese with antibiotics, cow milk with antibiotics, and ice cream with antibiotics—and they all have a touch of hormones.

Are these cows really healthy? What do you think?

According to Dr. Henri Joyeux, an oncologist and digestive surgeon, he does not recommend drinking any milk. He says the calcium from the animal is absorbed maximally by the gut at only about 40%. The remaining 60% is found in your waste. Calcium from plants, on the other hand, is absorbed up to 75%. Therefore, it is best to choose vegetables, especially organic, as your calcium source.

No hormones or antibiotics are part of the growing process, making them a healthier and more effective source of calcium. If you remember one of the worst things we can ingest is antibiotics that unbalance our intestinal flora. Also, vegetables are alkaline, which can help to balance out our acidity.

Today's diet is significantly more acidic than it was before. So, eat more alkaline foods.

That's not all! There are other problems related to milk. Some people have allergies or sensitivity to the milk protein, casein. Others also react to whey protein, while others have an inability to digest lactose, which is the milk sugar. Several people have a better tolerance for goat or sheep's milk. It is very important to take biological (organic), hormone-free, and antibiotic-free options. This can maximize the benefits, and lower the chances of an adverse reaction.

People with various health conditions (such as allergies, acne, sinus congestion, asthma, diabetes, digestive system problems, irritable bowel syndrome, osteoarthritis, rheumatoid arthritis, tendonitis, and immune problems), according to several testimonials, have seen improvement by banning cow products from their diets.

Instead, use fermented products, such as kefir. There are so many alternatives to cow's milk. You can drink vegetable (plant) milks, such as almond milk, cashew milk, coconut milk, hemp milk, and Brazil nut milk. The best is really to do it yourself. It's so easy! Just combine 2 ingredients: your nuts and water, before adding a touch of maple syrup, raw honey or stevia for taste and flavor, and even vanilla. You can ask for the recipe on sparknflynow.com.

Trying this could have benefits that make both your mind and body happy in the long run. This milk alternative is just one more step on your path to joining the epidemic of healthy people!

Is milk as good for you as they pretend it is in the commercials? You decide, but it might be worth considering a break from dairy products to see how much better you can feel.

SUGAR Loves CANCER!

Have you ever heard that we all have a cancer that sleeps within us?

Dr. Servan-Schreiber, who wrote the book, *Anticancer*, says: "Cancer feeds on sugar." He is not only the one who is saying this, as many holistic medicine doctors have been proclaiming this for a long period of time.

Today, we know the negative impacts of sugar, including weight gain, tooth decay, diabetes, and heart disease. But sugar also plays an important role in the development of cancer.

It is the German biologist, Otto Heinrich Warburg, that we owe for the discovery that the metabolism of cancer cells is dependent on sugar.

Do you know the PET SCAN? If you have known people with cancer, you are probably familiar with this particular test. This diagnostic tool can detect cancer in your body. How? By measuring the areas of your body that consume the most glucose, essentially sugar. If you have an area where there is an excessive consumption of glucose, it is likely that you have cancer.

So, they inject you with sugar to see if you have cancer! We know very well that cancer cells are more sensitive to glucose. They love glucose. So, why don't they tell you to reduce or stop your sugar intake when you have cancer? Why don't they advise you that sugar will impede your fight in healing your cancer? The answer is *money*, plain and simple.

Sugar consumption has drastically increased over the past few decades. Why is this the case? The food industry puts sugar into almost everything, even inside salty foods. This hidden sugar is nourishing cancer cells, all the while making the rest of your body work even harder to fight the destruction caused by sugar.

Sugar therefore feeds cancer cells!

The pancreas has to secrete insulin if you want the sugar to be absorbed by cells. This secretion is accompanied by the release of insulin-like growth factor-1 (IGF-1), a molecule which, in turn, participates in the growth of cancer cells and their invasion of the surrounding tissues.

The IGF also increases inflammation. You read earlier that inflammation is the basis of degenerative diseases, such as cancer.

Sugar is a food with a high index and glycemic load (wheat flour, corn syrup, wheat flour bread, instant rice, sugary cereals, wheat pasta, pastries, etc.), which stimulates much of your insulin production. It has the potential to create an ideal environment for the growth of cancer cells! These foods are found mainly on the shelves of your local grocery store!

Our modern diet is hyper PROCANCER!

What can help you? Consume foods with low glycemic index, such as organic fruits and vegetables, preferably those with a lot of fiber. Use and cook with coconut oil. Take a multivitamin of the highest quality, with a large spectrum of antioxidants, minerals, trace elements, and phytonutrients, manufactured by holding to a pharmaceutical standard and a guarantee of efficiency, purity, potency, and bioavailability.

Additionally, make sure that you are getting enough omega 3 that balances the ratio of omega 6 and 3, and thus reduces inflammation.

Finally, and most importantly, clean out your pantry to eliminate refined and processed foods, and replace them with healthy alternatives. When I say healthy, you need to pay attention to the food industry that uses labels, such as lighter, healthy choices, and best choice, to mislead the consumer about their health benefits. **They do not really care about your health. Business is business!**

When you run out of time to eat or cook, there are alternatives, such as well-balanced smoothies, but they are rare! You have to read the labels to know what you are getting.

Reduce your exposure to various toxins as much as possible. A very interesting book that can help you to do this is called *The Healthy Home.*

Cancer is a disease largely due to your lifestyle. What you do now, what you eat, breathe, drink, put on your skin, your activity level, your way of thinking, and your stress management has a direct impact on your future health. That is why you must not wait until tomorrow to make changes in your life but get started right now.

You have two choices: HEALTH or DISEASE.

There is no middle ground. Health is not merely the absence of visible signs of illness. Health is happening inside you. It is working. It is feeding.

If you are aware of all the information I have given you, then it should motivate you into action.

ACTIONS = RESULTS
DIFFERENT ACTIONS = DIFFERENT RESULTS

As Albert Einstein put it so well: *"Insanity is doing the same thing over and over again, and expecting different results."*

Are you ready to make a change? If you are not entirely convinced, then read on.

Is it Really Food?

Have you ever asked yourself if what you eat are real foods? Are you able to put an image in your head of the ingredients included in your food purchased at the grocery store?

For example, bread should contain how many ingredients?

The answer should be 4 or 5: flour, water, salt, yeast or leaven. Why do you find all kinds of ingredients in your food that you are unable to picture in your head?

What is the lifespan of a bread? A few days typically, but grocery bread can last weeks. Do you believe that this is normal for a food source that is supposedly natural and good for us?

Why are so many manufacturers adding ingredients in their bread, when bread should contain 4 or 5 ingredients at most? The majority of the surplus ingredients are called food additives.

What exactly is a food additive? An additive is something that is added to a food to improve the taste and color but also to increase the life of the food in question, reduce production costs, and increase the manufacturer's profits.

However, numerous scientific studies have established links between the use of these additives and various pathological conditions, such as cancer, diabetes, epidemic obesity, Alzheimer's, ADHD, and attention deficit disorders.

We are already bombarded by all chemical products and pollution in our environment, and then they add all these additives. When our grandparents were younger, they didn't have all the additives that we have today. But the additives are just a portion of the problem—you have to look at the artificial flavors.

Do you like chocolate? Who does not like that? Artificial chocolate flavor often has such a similar taste that we don't even know it isn't chocolate. They can make us eat anything! Chocolate flavoring and perfumes are used to mask a base product that might not taste good. When you see a label, for example, with chocolate flavoring or artificial chocolate flavor, just put it back on the shelf.

Flavor enhancers are added to enhance the perceived taste of a variety of products. They can make a tasty product out of bland and tasteless food. The reason is that they rely on stimulating parts of the brain to make us want to eat these products. One of the most common, the MONOSODIUM Glutamate (MSG), greatly improves the taste of food, and excites our brains! It is why MSG is used in the *fast food* industry and is very popular in Asian restaurants. We can also find MSG in many processed foods. A study from the *Journal of Autoimmunity* discovered that injection of MSG to mice causes inflammation in the liver, obesity, and type 2 diabetes. There are a variety of studies on the harmful effects of MSG.

According to Arizona Center for Advanced Medicine, MSG is blamed for a range of serious neurological and physiological disorders. Studies have identified MSG as excitotoxins, which are substances that overstimulate the neurotransmitters to the point of cell damage. Do you want to eliminate MSG from your diet? That may be harder than you think, as it is found in a large number of products.

According to Arizona Center for Advanced Medicine, **MSG shows up in:**

- Natural Flavorings
- Bouillon Cubes
- Hydrolyzed Vegetable Protein
- Hydrolyzed Plant Protein
- Autolyzed Plant Protein
- Sodium Caseinate
- Calcium Caseinate
- Textured Protein
- Yeast Extract
- Autolyzed Yeast
- Vegetable Protein Extract
- Gelatin
- Hydrolyzed Soy Protein
- E621
- And more…

Do you enjoy your morning coffee that you picked up in your favorite restaurant, service station, or coffee shop on the way to work? Well, that favorite coffee probably contains MSG. Why do you think you are so addicted to this coffee? It is better if you prepare your coffee at home and, preferably, choose organic options.

The famous MSG, this white powder that looks so harmless, is perhaps the worst food additive of the industry and is found in so many fast food and processed foods.

What About Artificial Sweeteners?

One of the best-known is ASPARTAME. It is still present in many foods. However, many studies show its excitotoxicity and its ability to disturb serotonin production.

Serotonin is also called the HORMONE OF HAPPINESS. It sounds good to your ears, doesn't it? Who does not search for HAPPINESS? This hormone, so important and essential, is involved in regulating circadian, sleep, and various disorders such as aggressiveness, stress, anxiety, depression, eating, and even sexual behavior. You can see how this hormone is so AMAZING!

There is not only aspartame, there are also other artificial sweeteners, such as acesulfame potassium, sucralose as *Splenda*, saccharin, and cyclamate. These are alternatives to the sugar that gives the sweet taste, without the calories. As they are artificial, how does our brain really perceive them? As a foreign body that would ignite your immune system? How do you think the brain processes them? Read the food labels! And don't touch them!

Do not forget your children. How do you think that all these additives affect their brain during development? Do you realize that they are growing up in a different environment than the one we did? Many young people today suffer increasingly from allergies, food intolerances, learning disabilities, attention deficits, ADHD, autism, and more. Start making changes every day by gradually eliminating these harmful substances to combat the negative impacts on your children.

Pay attention to many business products and supplements using these additives in their meal replacement shakes and bars, but also in their supplements for a pre or post workout. Aromas, flavors, colorants, and artificial sweeteners are included in their list of ingredients but written in small print on the label! They attract you with CARBS, PROTEINS, FATS, AMINO ACIDS, BCAA'S, MINERALS, and VITAMINS, so you often forget to check the list for hidden ingredients.

Instead, choose natural sugars, such as maple syrup and raw honey, or a small amount of the new stevia. BUT BE CAREFUL! Some companies attract you by mentioning the word Stevia, but behind that marketing tactic hides other ingredients, such as sucralose and other artificial sweeteners!

There are a multitude of food additives, and I invite you to start reading the labels! You and your family will feel better as you start making decisions based on the ingredients involved.

In our world today, it is almost impossible not to be tempted by the attractive packaging and boxes. The daily train of life runs continuously. You are busy and short on time.

Restaurants become the alternative to eating at home — multinationals that you know very well — with yummy burgers containing preservatives, texture agents, dyes, artificial flavors, MSG, antibiotics, and antimicrobial chemicals, some of which are also used in the metallurgical, cosmetic, and plastic industries. This is just to name a few. Isn't it strange that some foods do not rot? Normally, fresh and natural foods will eventually rot if they are not consumed quickly. Even the foods that they mention are healthier can have these chemical additions.

Finally, all refined and processed foods could trigger long-term diseases and create your inflammation, as well as reactions of all kinds.

Bring gradual changes into your life and consume nutritional supplements of the highest quality (see Chapter 1) with a large spectrum of antioxidants, minerals, trace elements, and phytonutrients, to protect you from these additives that are often hidden in your food without your knowledge.

Your cells need to be fed optimally, completing what is missing in your daily diet, being protected from all these damaging substances and being properly renewed.

Chapter 4

WHY ARE YOU MOVING?

Is it so Beneficial?

Yes, it is proven that moving is one of the pillars to achieve optimal health! Numerous scientific studies confirm this by studying activity levels in adults and children. The benefits cannot be overstated, and here are just a few to keep in mind the next time you want to put off going to the gym or taking that walk around the neighborhood.

Regarding overall health:

- Increased general energy level
- Improved sleep
- Improving your shape
- Regularization of appetite
- Optimizing your metabolism
- Feelings of well-being

Regarding physical and physiological health:

- Reduction of heart attack risk
- Increase *good* cholesterol (HDL)
- Decrease in blood pressure
- Improvement of the immune system
- Increased muscle mass
- Improved bone density
- Improved posture and balance

At the level of brain and mental health:

- Contribution to the brain and mental health
- Ability of neurons to modify their synaptic connections
- Neuroplasticity (new contact between neurons): learning
- Protection against neurodegeneration
- Reduced risk of developing Alzheimer's disease
- Improved blood flow
- Increased various neurotransmitters (including serotonin and endorphins)
- Better control of stress and anxiety

The benefits are endless, and yet many people remain sedentary or exercise infrequently. It then becomes a vicious cycle, because they don't feel good, so they don't exercise or get up and move. That makes them feel worse, and so they keep refraining from physical activity. It becomes a downward spiral, away from the health epidemic to one of chronic disease and ongoing health issues.

Beyond just keeping your muscles moving and giving you a healthy dose of endorphins, exercise has an even more important job, one that you wouldn't expect! Physical exercise is designed to **clean your sewers**!

Clean Your Sewers!

It may sound strange, but I'll explain it to you. The human body is composed of a heap of cells. All the tissues of your body, whether your organs (such as liver, intestines, heart, etc.), your soft tissues (such as skin, ligaments, tendons, etc.), your teeth, cartilage, or your bones, are composed of cells. In fact, you are made of trillions of them. These cells have multiple processing centers within them for digesting nutrients, releasing energy, and, of course, creating waste.

We could say that your cells resemble microscopic living creatures that continually work to maintain harmony in your body, depending on your lifestyle.

For your cells to function, they must live in two fluids: blood and lymph. The blood can feed and provide nutrients to your cells through the heart and lungs. Your cells must be fed properly. They must also eat and drink, just like you do. Your cells work and also create cellular waste as part of that process. That waste must be eliminated!

Waste from your cells are eliminated in the lymph, which bathes your cells. The lymph is actually the SEWER SYSTEM of YOUR CELLS!

There is more lymph than blood in your body because of the importance of elimination of your waste. Lymph contains no red blood cells, which is why it is rather colorless.

Blood flows because of your beautiful organ, the heart, pumping the blood through your arteries to ensure that your cells are nourished. That is why it is important to have good blood pressure to ensure that blood flows everywhere. Whether you are moving or not, the heart is making sure the blood is pumping.

But the lymph needs movement to circulate, because there is no distinct muscle, like the heart, for moving it throughout your body. Remember that well!

LYMPH = NEEDS MOVEMENT

If you sit all day in front of your computer, or you stay crashed on your couch, then the lymph does not circulate, or it does, but minimally at best.

You now understand the importance of moving your body, your muscles, and your joints, and doing it every day! By contracting your muscles, you stimulate your lymph so that it plays its role in disposal!

Did you know that the lymphatic system contains nodes? The nodes are tiny little organs that filter the lymphatic system. They clean the lymph and lymphocytes (a type of white blood cell) to remove cell waste, bacteria, viruses, foreign bodies, and more. In addition to this, they manufacture and store your cells that fight infection: lymphocytes. It is important, don't you think? The lymphatic system is an integral part of your IMMUNE SYSTEM!!!

These critical nodes are stimulated by the contraction of your muscles. If you are not active, you live with your waste, your filth! So how do you improve your health with all this dirt being left inside you?

Think about your small cells that are bathed in sewage. Do you think they like it? Would you like to be continually in sewage?

You need to be active! Your cells will thank you. The more lymph circulates, the more your cells are bathed in a liquid cleaner, as waste is carried away from your cells and disposed of.

Where do you think that this cellular waste is sent? To your intestines, where you find your food and cellular waste. How you feel and your mood, for example, can be the result of how your cells feel! If you are depressed, it is highly possible that your cells are bathed in a dirty liquid because your lymph can't do its job effectively.

BE ACTIVE FOR YOUR CELLS IF YOU WANT THEM TO BE HAPPY; AND THEREFORE, YOU WILL FEEL HAPPIER AND HEALTHIER!

Do You Need Supplements if You Train?

I have mentioned how the micronutrients (vitamins, minerals, antioxidants, and trace elements) are essential in the context of the life in which we live. Know that it is also very important for all sports and athletes. Nutrition is crucial to achieve the desired performance level. It allows the body to function well and meet the physiological needs of your cells every day. Sport brings many benefits to the body. However, paradoxically, did you know that it contributes to the production of free radicals? That damage causes premature aging of your cells. Daily, you face a multitude of free radicals, such as pollution, stress, pesticides, processed foods, secondhand smoke, Wi-Fi, electromagnetic waves, and chemicals in water, land, and air. You must then turn to nutrition to support your body in dealing with these damaging free radicals.

The nutrition is therefore the key, but the reality today is quite different. As I mentioned earlier, we are faced with poor nutritional quality.

In 2004, a research team in biochemistry from the University of Texas, led by Dr. Donald Davis, analyzed a report from the U.S. Department of Agriculture, for 43 common fruits and vegetables. They found that almost half of the substances that contained good healthy minerals had lost nutritional values. The researchers suggested that these declines were explained by changes in cultivated varieties, in which there may be "trade-offs between yield and nutrient content."

Dr. Davis mentioned that his team had not assessed individual fruits and vegetables, but they discovered nutritional losses in the group. "When we consider them as a group, we found that 6 of 13 nutrients showed declines between 1950 and 1999," stated the report. Now, imagine what it is today!

Nutrients that had lost measurable nutrient elements were the protein, calcium, phosphorus, iron, riboflavin, and ascorbic acid[16].

According to data from the nutrients provided by the U.S. Department of Agriculture, broccoli calcium content, which averaged 12.9 milligrams per gram, in 1950, has declined to show an average of 4.4 milligrams per gram, in 2003!

According to Philippe Desbrosses, PhD in environmental sciences at the University of Paris VII, "After decades of crossbreeding, the food industry has selected the most beautiful vegetables and more resistant, but rarely the most nutritionally rich." The activist supports the preservation of ancient seeds.

How can you incorporate into your daily life all the nutritional considerations to maximize the health benefits, considering the changes to our food?

If we are missing nutrients inside our fruits and vegetables, logically then, we are living with deficiencies. We can't say that we have everything in our fruits and vegetables, because we don't. If you believe that we do, then you don't see the facts, or you are unwilling to face the reality!

I firmly believe, and it's supported by so many scientific studies, that supplementation should be part of our lives. Several scientific studies show the benefits of consuming a supplement with food for active people and those in sports, and more specifically for elite athletes and those who practice endurance sports, because they require greater antioxidant protection[17].

Here is an idea of what you need. This is really a short explanation but gives you a great overview of what these minerals, trace elements, vitamins, and antioxidants are used for.

Minerals and Trace Elements:

CALCIUM:
- Important for bone health, and many people do not know that it is essential for each muscle contraction.
- If the muscles are deficient in calcium, the body will

provide it by taking it from your bones. You don't want that!

MAGNESIUM:
- Essential to sports because when the muscles are relaxed, magnesium moves in muscle cells.
- If there is deficiency, the muscles cannot relax, and the individual may have muscle cramps.
- During physical activity, a lot of magnesium is lost through sweat and breathing.

ZINC:
- Participates in the synthesis of proteins, carbohydrates and fats, immune processes and wound healing.
- Involved in the blood clotting process
- Plays a role in the metabolism of insulin.
- Is very important in weight loss.

IODE:
- Indispensable for the production of thyroid hormones that regulate:
  * metabolism
  * growth
  * reproduction
  * protein synthesis
- Anti-microbial and anti-inflammatory role.
- Essential for heart health.

SELENIUM:
- Is a trace element of our system of internal defenses against free radicals.

- Also protects the immune system and has anti-inflammatory properties.

MANGANESE:
- Important cofactor in the development of glycosaminoglycans, compounds that form cartilages, connective tissues, bones, arteries, and other organs.

CHROME:
- Helps maintain a healthy glucose metabolism while assisting the body to metabolize carbohydrates and fats.
- Is very important in weight loss.

Many other minerals are important.

Vitamins:

COMPLEX B consists of 8 vitamins (B1, B2, B3, B5, B6, B8, B9, B12).

Vitamin B3 is produced in small but insufficient amounts by the body and vitamin B12, is stored in certain organs, including the liver. We must make up for the deficiency of these two vitamins and supply our body with other vitamins of the B complex by eating on a regular basis. Also these vitamins are rapidly eliminated in the urine. That is why they should be renewed on a daily basis.

B3 (niacin)
- Plays a key role in the extraction and use of energy from carbohydrates, proteins, and lipids.

B5 (pantothenic acid):
- Anti-stress vitamin that is stored in large amounts in the adrenal glands.

B6:
- Essential element for protein digestion, absorption, and metabolism of amino acids.
- It is most crucial to improving immune function

B9:
Involved:
- In the production of white and red blood cells
- Wound healing
- Protein metabolism

B12:
- Participates in the synthesis of red blood cells and nucleic acids (DNA and RNA).
- It plays a role in the effectiveness of the immune system.

The Famous VITAMIN C:
- Powerful antioxidant
- Important role in the synthesis of collagen (component of ligaments, tendons, bones, skin, etc.).
- Role in the synthesis of red blood cells (manufactured by bone marrow).
- Virtues: anti-fatigue, anti-infection, anti-histamine, anti-cancer....
- Promotes recovery after exercise.
- Improves lung capacity and reduces rapid heartbeat.
- Promotes the absorption of iron.

- Water-soluble vitamin (soluble in water), so it must be renewed every day.

VITAMIN E:
- Reduces the production of free radicals and reduces tissue damage.
- Has anti-inflammatory, antiplatelet, and vasodilator properties.
- Cardio-protective role.

BETA CAROTENE AND VITAMIN A:
- Role in the growth, repair, and cellular differentiation.
- BETA CAROTENE is a precursor of Vitamin A.

VITAMIN D:
- Vitamin miracle!
- Influences so many genes and has a DNA repair action.
- Enables faster recovery after exercise.
- Role in neuromuscular function.

VITAMINS (A, C, E):
- Fight against the formation of the free radicals linked to intense muscular activity.
- Also limit the inflammatory phenomena caused by micro-trauma, such as tendonitis and edema.

Several other vitamins also contribute to a variety of daily body functions.

Other Powerful Nutrients:

CoQ10 (coenzyme Q10):
- Coenzyme, which acts as a vitamin in the body, activates the production of energy on the cellular level. All physiological processes that require energy expenditure need CoQ10.
- Is found in greater numbers in the muscle cells of the heart. CoQ10 is essential in the process to burn sugars and fats and convert them into energy.
- * Know that CoQ10 levels decrease with age. That's why it can be very interesting to take it as a supplement if you are looking to increase your energy.

GRAPE SEED EXTRACT
- A powerful, natural antioxidant that has a role in anti-inflammatory and anti-pain on the body and helps in circulation.
- Studies show that when combined with vitamin C, the benefits are thereby multiplied.

CURCUMIN is a strong antioxidant, anti-inflammatory, and immunomodulatory.

RHODIOLA (rhodiola rosea) is an adaptogenic plant— that is to say it adapts to the needs of the organism. This plant would have many benefits.

- Increases energy
- Tones muscles
- Increases performance

- Boosts the immune system
- Helps the body to destroy toxins
- Help to stress adaptation level
- Allows a better tissue perfusion
- Normalizes the heartbeat after exercise
- Increase bioavailability of serotonin, which affects mood and the winter blues....

GLUCOSAMINE is an important element in maintaining the health of your joints. It is an important precursor for the production of cartilage, which is vital since it serves as a damper and prevents the bones from rubbing against each other. Unfortunately, with age, the cushioning diminishes, and our body is struggling to maintain healthy cartilage.

OMEGA 3 promotes soft tissue, improve lubrication in joints, and decrease the inflammatory reactions in the body. They increase the power reached at the end of a maximum stress test and help to transform the glycogen into energy. They are also very important for brain and nerve health.

Sports or not, although I recommend exercise and activity for those who are not involved in sports, you all need minerals, vitamins, antioxidants, and trace elements, to ensure optimum performance.

Even then, you have to choose the uncompromising quality when you optimize your health through supplementation!!!

---

[16] DAVIS, D., M.D. EPP et H.D. RIORDAN. «Changes in USDA Food Composition Data for 43 Garden Crops, 1950 to 1999», Journal of the American College of Nutrition, vol. 23, n° 6 (2004), p. 669-682.

[17] MacWilliam, Lyle, Msc. (2008) Suppléments nutritionnels. Northern Dimensions Publishing, p.12.

Chapter 5

WHY DO YOU NEED SLEEP TO BE HEALTHY?

D id you know that when you are 75 years old, you will have slept approximately for 25 years of your lifetime? Yes, it's true! This represents 1/3 of your life! But why do we sleep so much? Do you see this as a waste of time? Well, read this carefully to get a better appreciation for how critical sleep is!

Sleep is an extremely important pillar in assuring optimal health. In fact, it could be one of the most important parts of creating a health epidemic in your own life.

Sleeping is one of the most important factors in the reconstruction and consolidation of our immune system. Our immune system must be strong to fight against all bacteria, viruses, or foreign bodies. Do you sincerely believe that a cold will stick to you if your immune system is powerful? Of course not! With all the toxins in our environment and the poor quality of our food, we really have to do our best to help it.

One of the most important things is SLEEP! It's during slow and deep sleep that the body strengthens our white blood cells or leukocytes, which are really a pillar of our immune system. Have you noticed that people who are chronically sleep deprived are more prone to a host of infections? Studies confirm it. When we generally do not sleep well, because of various reasons, including stress, it's easier to get the flu or a cold. Many people have the false belief that it is normal to get the flu or a cold. The true reason is just that your immune system is weak and trying to fight. Imagine your army of little soldiers that are part of your immune system. When you are sick, we may imagine that some of them are sleeping or are lazy. Take two people who are in contact with a sick person who has a bad flu. Why does one of the two not contract this virus? After all, they have both been in contact with the virus. Are these soldiers stronger than the others? Perhaps his army is more powerful and numerous? Maybe, and it could be as simple as the amount of sleep each one is getting.

During sleep, our body manufactures and repairs our cells. It's during phases 3 and 4 of sleep that the body synthesizes most of its proteins. If you do not sleep well, how can you expect your body to succeed in mending itself?

That's not all. Sleep is also used to rebuild our mental strength. The brain benefits from sleep. This rest time is so precious to strengthen our neural circuits but also to produce new ones. There is a direct connection between our capacity for concentration and alertness during the day, and the quality of our sleep!

It's during the slow and REM sleep that the brain sorts out all what you have learned during your day. What will the brain keep and throw out? Several people have hallucinations and symptoms of mental illness when they are deprived of REM sleep for just a few days.

Experiments were performed on rats that were REM sleep deprived. These rats would die very quickly, while that was not the case when they were deprived of the other sleep stages. Insomnia can even accentuate a psychological disorder, and vice versa.

Virtually all our body systems take advantage of night time, for restoring, repairing, cleaning, recovering, and replenishing strength and energy. Indisputably, sleep is essential in the life of every living being!

DID YOU KNOW that sleep deficiency has been linked to a shorter life expectancy and a higher risk of developing a degenerative disease? Clearly, sleep is a key to a healthier lifestyle and for joining the epidemic of healthy people.

How can you improve your quality of sleep? It starts with making sure that you have the right hormones.

Melatonin: A RESTORATIVE HORMONE That You Need

Melatonin is a natural hormone produced by the pineal gland, located in the brain and barely the size of a pea! This hormone is secreted in response to the absence of light. It is best known as a hormone that plays a central role in the regulation of chronobiologic rhythms (cortisol, temperature, blood pressure, blood sugar, growth and development, reproduction, and so on). It is synthesized from the neurotransmitter, SEROTONIN, that famous happy hormone, which itself is derived from tryptophan. Therefore, we must produce enough serotonin to have enough melatonin! The two are intricately connected.

Melatonin also regulates many hormonal secretions among both humans and mammals. Do you know why hormones are so important? They are chemical messengers that are transported throughout the body. In general, hormones are sent via the bloodstream to one or more target organs in order to modify its operation by stimulating or inhibiting one of its functions.

Melatonin would also have a protective effect against the development and progression of cancer. In a study done on American nurses, those who worked night shifts for more than 30 years had a 36% higher risk of developing breast cancer[18].

According to Sanoviv Medical Institute, melatonin has antioxidant properties. By allowing the body to get sleep and rest, it allows our natural antioxidant defenses to counteract oxidative stress accumulated during the day. In addition, it stimulates the activity of several antioxidant enzyme systems in our body.

Melatonin production also stimulates the synthesis of immune cells, a process that naturally declines with age. Also, it plays an anti-inflammatory role, anti-thrombotic, and anti-blood lipids.

To benefit from the best conditions, during the day we have to be exposed to daylight, thus our melatonin is inhibited. At night, however, we have to be exposed to the darkness in order to secrete it.

To be part of the epidemic of healthy people, you need this wonderful hormone, MELATONIN.

It can be really interesting taking melatonin in supplement form. However, you must ensure purity. The primary advantage is that it does not cause addiction, as does some sleep medications. It should contain a guarantee of potency, purity, efficiency, and safety, and follow pharmaceutical grade.

In addition, if you suffer from poor sleep and you're struggling to calm down your body and head at night time, you surely need magnesium.

Magnesium : Our Natural Muscle Relaxant

According to a study, the dietary intake in magnesium is insufficient in 60% of the North American population[19]. This statistic varies with geographic location, but the implication is clear that for a majority of us, we aren't getting enough magnesium.

Magnesium is an essential mineral, and yet it constitutes only about 0.05% of our total body weight. It is an important component to maintain strong and healthy bones. It participates in more than 300 metabolic reactions in the body! This mineral works closely with sodium, potassium, and calcium, with which it must remain in balance. It is so important that I could write about it for pages and pages. However, here I want to focus on its natural muscle relaxant properties. It plays a leading role in neuromuscular contractions. We are compounds of about 600 muscles, and they must be able to contract and relax. Magnesium allows relaxation after muscle contraction.

Imagine that your biceps are constantly in contraction! Ouch!!! Would you be able to properly eat a meal? Of course not! Your arm would be constantly tired.

Now imagine you are sleeping, and the muscles of your face are constantly contracted! Do you believe that your sleep will be disturbed?

Imagine that you run, and your quadriceps, which allow the extension of your legs, remain contracted! Will you be able to keep running? With these images, it's easy understanding how important magnesium truly is.

We have a variety of muscles that let us eat, smile, and move! Your heart is also made up of muscles. Imagine, if your heart never relaxed and always stayed contracted. There would be no blood flow throughout the body. Now you understand how vital magnesium is!

Did you know that a simple blood test does not allow you to properly assess your amount of magnesium[20]? Only about 1% of magnesium in our bodies is in our blood. The magnesium levels in the blood may be adequate despite very deficient reserves. Your blood being rich or poor in magnesium does not indicate that your cells and tissues are rich or poor in magnesium.

It's really difficult to find the right amount of magnesium in our diet, so it is really vital to take this mineral in supplements. Again, we must choose the best one. You can see my recommendations in Chapter 1.

Stop being tense. Instead, feel relaxed and calm with magnesium!

[18] J National Cancer Institute 17 Oct 2001- Nurses who worked night shifts had a higher risk of breast cancer.

[19] Tucker KL. Dietary Intake and Bone Status with Aging. Curr Pharm Des 2003 ;9:2687-2704.

[20] Elin RJ. Assessment of magnesium status for diagnosis and therapy. Magnes Res 2010;23:1-5. [PubMed abstract]

Pillar 2 :
MIND

Chapter 6

DOES YOUR BRAIN
PLAY TRICKS ON YOU?

Can Food Affect Your Brain?

W hen we talk about the notion of health, it is impossible to put aside the biochemistry of our brain. Our brain and its many functions play a significant role in how we feel and take care of ourselves. An ill-fed brain would have an impact on the entire body!

In this magnificent machine, which is our brain, there are extremely important chemical messengers: the neurotransmitters. These will create important changes on our way of thinking, our mood, our feelings, and thus affect the way we interact with others. They can affect our sleep, our memory, our energy, our self-confidence, and our metabolism ... in fact, all our systems!

Without neurotransmitters, the brain could not communicate with the rest of the body! Without them, we would be incapable of seeing, thinking, hearing, touching, feeling, tasting, understanding, and experiencing feelings and emotions.

Now you understand their importance! So, knowing this, we have every interest in not having any missing neurotransmitters! So, where do we find them?

Some neurotransmitters come directly from our daily diet!

As you have learned before, we face significant short-comings in our everyday diet. Given the poor quality of modern foods, these shortcomings are INEVITABLE. Refining, denaturation by adding chemical additives, processed foods, deficient cultivation methods, use of chemical fertilizers, pesticides and other chemicals, pollution, methods of collection, transport, storage, cooking, and more, all contribute to these shortcomings. We need a better understanding of the causes of deficient nutritional intake in our food today.

Nutritional supplements exist to meet our FUNDAMENTAL NEED for good nutrition. They are essential to anyone who wants to avoid nutritional deficiencies.

What Are the Essential Nutrients for Our Brain?

The brain, the body's fattest organ, requires high-quality fats, such as **OMEGA 3.** These fats, derived from fish oil and certain plants, have important functions in the brain, such as controlling inflammation due to immune reactions, helping eliminate free radicals, changing nerve transmissions, and altering brain cells.

Moreover, we must not forget that our brain is composed of cells like all the rest of our body. Each cell is formed of a biphospholipid membrane, whose flexibility and fluidity depend on its ratio of OMEGA. Thus, by having a well-balanced ratio in omega 3, and 6, the transmissions of the nerve impulses and the exchanges at the cellular level are optimized. As we saw earlier, today's diet is deficient in omega 3. We should not ask why we have so many cognitive problems, cases of depression, mood swings, fatigue, discomfort, brain diseases, and so on.

To address this deficiency, consume small fish, such as sardines, anchovies, and mackerel, but do not forget to add a supplement of an omega 3 capsule, certified WITHOUT HEAVY METALS! You can also add omega 3 oils from plants (flax, hemp, pumpkin, etc.). However, be aware that you will need to consume more from plants, especially if you do not consume omega 3 from a marine source, since they are not already processed into EPA (eicosapentaenoic acid) and DHA (docosahexaenoic acid), which are the active compounds of Omega 3. In addition, you will need to make sure that your liver has the ability to transform them.

A simple increase in OMEGA 3 could make a difference in the health of your brain!

Do not forget to care for yourself!!!

Do not forget to use supplements WITHOUT HEAVY METALS!

ANTIOXIDANTS are also very protective for the brain. The role of antioxidants is to neutralize the free radicals that damage our cells. However, did you know that you have a blood-brain barrier? The role of this barrier is to isolate the brain from unwanted substances that may end up in the bloodstream. It separates the brain from the blood. It makes it difficult to pass the nutrients to the cells, except those that play an indispensable role in the functioning of the brain. It is important to have enough antioxidants that pass through this barrier in order to have a positive impact on our brain.

VITAMIN E succeeds in crossing the barrier, but with a certain degree of difficulty.

VITAMIN C is an excellent antioxidant and has the ability to regenerate vitamin E and glutathione.

GLUTATHIONE is difficult to absorb in oral form. It would probably be more beneficial to give the body the nutrients it needs to make its own glutathione (N-acetyl L-cysteine, niacin, selenium, vitamin B2) and antioxidants to regenerate it (vitamin C, alpha lipoic acid, and CoQ10).

ALPHA-LIPOIC ACID (water-soluble and fat-soluble at the same time). It also has the ability to regenerate vitamin C, vitamin E, intracellular glutathione, and CoQ10! It would also have the ability to attach to the toxic metals found in the brain and help eliminate them from the body. Wow!

COENZYME Q10 (one of the most important cellular energy producing nutrients). Know that the level of CoQ10 in our brain, nerve cells, and all the cells in our body decreases considerably with age.

GRAPE SEED EXTRACT (exceptionally powerful and effective antioxidant for crossing the barrier). It would be interesting to have more studies done on it.

GINKGO BILOBA (improves blood circulation to the brain).

We face an increasingly toxic environment. Antioxidants contribute to the proper functioning of the brain and provide protection against neurodegenerative diseases.

Never forget that your brain must feed and protect itself to ensure its ability to perform its many vital functions! The better it is fed, the more it will give you in ENERGY and VITALITY, which will give you BETTER PERFORMANCE!

Does the Food You Eat Play with Your Emotions?

Food is very often used to help us *deal* with stress or emotional pain. Have you ever eaten a good chunk of chocolate cake to make you feel better or because you just feel the need? Or maybe, it is a good bag of chips or some other sort of treat? Unfortunately, this behavior of yielding to temptation manifests how your brain is manipulated in a bad way.

Many people choose comforting foods in the moment, which bring immediate gratification, but in the long run, these foods bring dull moods, low energy levels, loss of vitality, fatigue, and even exhaustion.

Many suffer from biochemical imbalance in the brain and body because of their diet. The agri-food industry has changed so much. Sugar, *fast food*, bad fats, food additives, colors, flavors, artificial sweeteners, preservatives, and salts are part of the daily lives of a majority of people. Add to this a lack of exercise, stress, lack of time, media pressure, and a lack of sleep, which is part of our lifestyle, and you have the causes of biochemical imbalances that will affect our behavior and our health! Do you realize this?

It is important to know that every bite of food you consume breaks down in your digestive system into small molecules that bring information that will be good or erroneous to the cells in your body and your brain. This information may, therefore, be favorable or not favorable to your health. It is very important to be aware of this.

Without awareness, there is no change!

Does Your Blood Sugar Level Affect Your Brain?

Blood sugar, which represents the level of sugar in our blood, is one of the things that can affect the biochemistry of our brain. Do you remember Chapter 2 where I explained the notion of the glycemic index? The more a food has a high glycemic index, the faster it will increase the level of sugar in our blood. We also need to take into account the notion of glycemic load, which is the amount of carbohydrates in the food. However, in general, the glycemic index gives a very good idea of our blood sugar levels.

I told you that when you eat these high-glycemic foods, you always have a glycemic peak followed by a reactional hypoglycemia, which causes you to feel tired, with a lack energy and concentration, uncomfortable, sometimes irritable, and even aggressive. Your body detects that something is missing and tells you to feel that particular way. You want to get out of this state as quickly as possible. What are you going to do? Consume another high carbohydrate food (with high glycemic index), which will give you temporary false energy (because of the sugar)! You will experience a rollercoaster of sugar highs and lows!

Have you noticed that during more stressful periods, accompanied by lack of sleep and an increased workload, you have more periods of *craving*, or sugar rages? At this point, you will be more likely to eat these high-sugar content foods! Do you really believe that they help you to restart your biochemistry and regain your energy? Not at all! They create even more imbalance! A true INFERNAL CYCLE!!!

Serotonin Imbalance

If you present a biochemical imbalance, there are foods and supplements that can support the increase in specific neurotransmitters, and restore balance. I have already spoken to you about SEROTONINE, one of the powerful hormones that is also called the famous HORMONE OF HAPPINESS. This is manipulated each day by the type of food we consume.

Again, I feel the need to mention it. If you have sufficient serotonin levels, you will tend to feel happier with yourself, more confident, more satisfied, and have a good level of well-being. However, when your levels are low, you may feel depressed, unwell, and have an intense rage for sugar, alcohol, and starchy foods. You actually will feel the need to consume them. In the long run, you will gain weight, have insatiable rages, and may even have a pessimistic and depressive attitude.

Serotonin is made from the amino acid, TRYPTO-PHANE, which comes from the proteins we consume. However, it is very important to know that eating tryptophan-rich foods does not increase serotonin systematically. This amino acid finds itself in competition with the other amino acids to be absorbed by the blood circulation! Foods, such as turkey, chicken, nuts, eggs, salmon and other fish, quinoa, avocados, legumes and bananas, can help you increase your level of serotonin. Eating essential fatty acids, like OMEGA 3, would also have an effect on the functioning of serotonin in the brain.

Personally, I consume daily supplements of omega 3, with a guarantee of purity, and certified without heavy metals. Flee like the plague from omega 3 supplements that do not guarantee purity! Heavy metals, such as mercury, arsenic, and lead, are contained in a large majority of omega 3 supplements, and they cross the blood-brain barrier of the brain! They damage your brain!!! How illogical!

Get moving! According to Marc Belisle, a professor in sports psychology at the Faculty of Physical Education and Sports at the University of Sherbrooke, physical activity promotes the proper functioning of neurotransmitters. Studies have shown that physical activity is a more effective treatment than antidepressants, particularly for mild to moderate depression, the latter accounting for 2/3 of cases of depression diagnosed in Quebec, Canada. Also, it does not cause side effects. Studies have shown that after one year, there have been more relapses of depression with antidepressants than with physical activity[21]. Do you think it's different elsewhere in the world? Probably not!

The sun and light would probably help the synthesis of serotonin.

According to Mayo clinic, decreased sun exposure has been associated with a drop-in serotonin that can lead to SAD (Season Affective Disorder).

Get outdoors!!!

We have every interest in increasing our level of SEROTONINE to live a life full of happiness!

Can Food Make You Addicted?

Yes, no doubt, there is also DEPENDENCE in food. We are familiar with addictions to alcohol, cigarettes, drugs, and medications.

However, did you know that food addiction also exists? The need for a substance or food is a certain form of dependence. Not being able to say no, and needing certain food or a substance to calm down and relax, while knowing that it is damaging to you, is truly addictive! This addiction can really sabotage your health and your quality of life!

So why do some people consume it anyway?

First, we must begin by realizing that food can create a dependency on the same level as alcohol dependence. Be aware that certain types of foods are really addictive. So, this is a first step to bring you toward a positive change.

WITHOUT CONSCIOUS EFFORT, NO CHANGE IS POSSIBLE!

A processed food, which is no longer in its natural state and has undergone various transformations, is more likely to be *addictive* than a food in its natural state. Take, for example, these famous energy drinks or soft drinks. How many people consume this type of drink and cannot do without them? Do you really know what these drinks contain and what damage they can create to your body? For those who do not consume soft drinks, then take the example of bread. We are very far from the bread of the past with its 3–4 ingredients! It makes no sense anymore! Look carefully at the bread you eat and count the number of ingredients on the label.

Here are the questions you need to ask:

- How many ingredients does it contain?
- Do you have a clear understanding of each of the ingredients?
- Does it contain sugars?
- How long will it stay fresh?

The fact that it contains many ingredients, that you do not get a clear picture of these, and that the bread lasts more than a week, proves that's it's a completely transformed food, which may cause you to become addicted and have other health problems.

A study from Neuroscience and Biobehavioral Reviews states that we can be addicted to sugar the same way we can be to heroin, cocaine, or nicotine[22]! Terrifying, no? Controlled by sugar!

The worst is that the food industry knows very well what makes foods so addictive and attractive. Yes, you heard right! That's why they insert certain substances in most processed foods to stimulate our brain! They know very well that they have a biochemical effect in our brain, making us even more inclined to consume them!

Now you understand how much your BRAIN can change its biochemistry through food!!! Your food controls you and influences you! You have an interest in choosing and consuming the right foods!

Take conscious action in order to bring about changes; because unconscious behavior has no chance in causing you to change!!! Hopefully, this book will bring you to think and better understand the urgency of making better food choices!

Where Should You Start?

Ready! I suggest that you COMMIT to making changes, one step at a time, and talking to a positive friend about it. Sharing will push you more into making changes, to committing yourself, and above all to keeping your commitment. During my coaching and lectures, I pay particular attention to the WHY. You need to discover the WHY that motivates you to change. Above all, write down all the reasons that make it important for you. The more reasons, the greater your chance of success! Then, put them clearly in sight in different parts of your home (bedroom, kitchen, living room, work desk, and even on your computer screen, and cell phone). Then, direct your attention and your mindset on this WHY. Your results (which you currently have) are no coincidence! They are the accumulation of choices you have made so far in your life. By focusing on your WHY, you will focus at the same time on the results you want to achieve.

Tips:

- At every meal, eat high-quality protein and fibers, with a guarantee of purity and assimilation, which will help you to be better supported.
- Listen more to the signals your body sends you. Be sensitive to drops in energy levels and find out which foods brought you to this state. YOUR BODY SPEAKS TO YOU! You should listen to it!!! Do not wait until you're in the hospital emergency room before deciding to change!
- Cut soft drinks, energy drinks, grocery juices, and even juices that do not contain fiber.
- Avoid artificial sweeteners, artificial flavors, and artificial colors.
- Consume more foods that are in their natural state and, therefore, unprocessed.
- Cook!

- Get back in touch with yourself. Make appointments with yourself every week and, above all, put them on your agenda.
- Reward yourself with a good massage, or an alternative medicine treatment! Pamper yourself!
- Have a partner you can count on. They can be called your partner to whom you are indebted. Call each other every day at a specific time, and take less than 5 minutes to update your progress! You can tell him your good choices of the day! It will help you stay accountable for your decision in changing how you eat and move.
- If you need help, Spark N Fly and I can actually help you with our different wellness programs, plus step by step guides to help you in obtaining your goals.
- Visit sparknflynow.com!

Do Nutritional Supplements Influence Your Brain?

Nutritional supplements work, like drugs, hormones, and foods, on a biochemical scale. They can provide energy, allow chemical reactions, act as enzymes, cofactors, and also help to reconstitute a missing or insufficient element.

Essential minerals (calcium, magnesium, zinc, iodine, copper, selenium, manganese, potassium, sodium, phosphorous, chromium, molybdenum, cobalt, iron, silicon, sulfur, etc.), essential vitamins (A, B1, B2, B3, B5, B6, B8, B9, B12, C, D, E, K), CoQ10, alpha lipoic acid, and essential fatty acids, like omega 3, are really important and can have an effect on your brain, especially when you have an insufficient quantity in your body.

Imagine an assembly line for automotive design. If, at the end of the chain, some elements were absent, do you think your car would work to its full potential? It may be drivable for a time, but eventually, it no longer will. Your body is the vehicle that you will have all your life. Cell production and renewal occur every day. If you run out of energy or have a health problem, then chances are you are missing essential items.

The environment in which we live (PCBs, chemical agents in water, earth and air, pesticides, waves of any kind, microwave, WIFI, oil and nuclear wastes, non-stick pans with aluminum or other substances, etc.) also affect the biochemistry of our brain.

Did you know that nearly 143,000 chemicals have been listed globally[23]?

Here is a study from the American Journal of Clinical Nutrition that focused on patients hospitalized in intensive care. These patients received 500 mg of vitamin C, twice daily, and 5000 IU of vitamin D per day.

CONCLUSION: Short-term therapy with vitamin C improves mood and reduces psychological distress in acutely hospitalized patients with a high prevalence of hypovitaminosis C and D. No conclusion is possible regarding the effects of vitamin D, because the dose and duration of therapy were insufficient to raise 25 (OH) D concentrations into the normal range[24].

In the January 2015 issue of *The Lancet Psychiatry*, an international team, led by Dr. Jerome Sarris, found a relationship between diet quality and potential nutritional deficiencies and mental health.

Studies show that many of these nutrients have a clear link to brain health, including omega-3s, B vitamins (particularly folate and B12), choline, iron, zinc, magnesium, S-adenosyl methionine (SAMe), vitamin D, and amino acids.

"While we advocate for these to be consumed in the diet where possible, additional select prescription of these as nutraceuticals (nutrient supplements) may also be justified," Dr. Sarris said. "While the determinants of mental health are complex, the emerging and compelling evidence for nutrition as a key factor in the high prevalence and incidence of mental disorders suggests that nutrition is as important to psychiatry as it is to cardiology, endocrinology, and gastroenterology[25]."

You probably have a better understanding of why nutritional deficiencies should be avoided as much as possible! Nutritional supplements definitely have an important role to play in maintaining a biochemical balance in our brain, given the context of life today!

Does Stress Affect Your Brain?

Every human being, during his/her life, will undergo various stresses in different areas (work, couple, family, friends, finances, physical and mental health, diseases, etc.).

It is important to distinguish between acute and chronic stress. For example, if you are a victim of a fire, you must be able to react quickly! Your heart rate and breathing are accelerating. The amount of blood sent to your muscles increases to make you move quickly. Your digestive system is slowed down, because it is not the time to digest your last meal. This is a normal stress, even ESSENTIAL! It is called acute stress.

However, when stress becomes chronic, it is a whole different story!! When it persists, then it is harmful and can really cause you to be vulnerable to disease.

One of the biggest repercussions of chronic stress is on the digestive system. Stress affects organs, especially the stomach by inhibiting the emptying of it. The stomach is thus unable to empty its contents. The motricity (peristalsis) of your small intestine is disrupted. Intestinal transit is affected at the colon. If these organs of the digestive system are disturbed, then a host of consequences are set in motion (poor digestion, poor absorption and assimilation of nutrients that can lead to malnutrition and nutritional deficiencies, poor elimination that can lead to constipation, toxin retention, intoxication, etc.).

Stress closes the doors of your digestive system!!!

I forgot to tell you about your brain! Stress could change your brain, your brain size, its structure, and how it functions, right down to the level of your genes. So, long-term stress ups your risk of brain disorders!

Precious Help to Reduce Stress

- Some nutritional supplements can greatly help. For example, taking vitamins B5–B6 can give good support to the adrenal glands.
- The rhodiola plant is an adaptogenic plant that could increase the body's resistance to stress factors, both chemical, physical, and biological.
- Magnesium is also considered a natural muscle relaxant.
- Take an array of antioxidants that can have an impact on oxidative stress.
- Activities, such as yoga, meditation, prayer, deep breathing exercises, and cardiac coherence, can be very helpful in bringing calm and relaxation.
- The morning routine can also be very useful. Following a good night's sleep, it is important to get anchored to focus on the priority objectives of the day.
- Never neglect your sleep! And respect the sleep cycles and the period when melatonin, the hormone of deep sleep, is most stimulated. It may be helpful to use melatonin additionally to help.
- Move because physical activity stimulates the production of endorphins!

- Consult an osteopath. The osteopath works at the level of the visceral organs, the craniosacral system, and the vegetative nervous system to rebalance their functions.
- And never forget to SMILE! Smiling automatically brings about a biochemical change in our body!

In sum, what you eat and drink, your level of physical activity, your sleep, your environment, the people around you, and the way you think and react to events, undoubtedly plays a part in the BIOCHEMISTRY of your brain!

In the context of today's life and the stress we face, nutritional supplements have their place.

Supplement your brain for optimal performance!

---

[21] Reference : www.santepratique.fr/serotonine-definition.php and Marc Bélisle, professor in sports psychology at the Faculty of Physical and Sports Education of the University of Sherbrooke.

[22] Neuroscience and Biobehavioral Reviews. 2008; 32 (1): 20-39. Epub 2007 May 18. Evidence for sugar addiction: behavioral and neurochemical effects of intermittent, excessive sugar intake. Avena NM1, Rada P, Hoebel BG.

[23] From document: PRE-POLLUTED: A REPORT ON THE TOXIC SUBSTANCES IN THE UMBILICAL CORD BLOOD OF CANADIAN NEWBORNS.

[24] Wang Y, Liu XJ, Robitaille L, Eintracht S, MacNamara E, Hoffer LJ. Effects of vitamin C and vitamin D on hospitalized patients. Am J Clin Nutr. 2013 Sep; 98 (3): 705-11. Doi: 10.3945 / ajcn.112.056366. PubMed PMID: 23885048.

[25] Rahilly A. Diet and nutrition essential for mental health. 28 January 2015. Medicalxpress, Psychology & Psychiatry. http://medicalxpress.com/news/2015-01-diet-nutrition-essential-mental-health.html.

Chapter 7

YOUR PERSONAL DEVELOPMENT TO A LEVEL YOU NEVER THOUGHT OF!

Your Energy Level

To be able to live a stimulating, extraordinary, happy life, you need ENERGY! Without energy, everything works in slow motion. So, to become energetic, nutrition and supplementation must be a PRIORITY! When energy is there, everything is possible! Your ideas are clearer, you can focus better on your goals, and thus be more productive and effective.

You only have to compare the following day after a night of insomnia, as opposed to a restful night. Which one left you the most productive, effective, and able to focus on your work? You know very well what the answer is! Without energy, everything moves at a much slower pace. Perhaps you are thinking: "I'm fine. I have plenty of energy!" Or you might be thinking, "I'm normal. I'm no longer that young."

Are you really sure? If high-quality supplementation is not part of your daily life to address your current nutritional deficiencies in the context of today's life, then I'm sorry to have to mention it again, but you are not fulfilling your FULL POTENTIAL!!! NOT POSSIBLE!

The energy level makes the difference! Would you prefer following an energetic person or an amorphous person? We are attracted by energy. It creates movement, action, efficiency, productivity, and change.

Change is a word that scares many people! Are we made to stagnate? Of course not! We were created to evolve—so, change! Why does the word, *change*, scare some people? I sincerely believe that one of the causes of fear of change comes from our beliefs!

Everything Begins with a Belief!

What is a belief? It's something you believe. For example, you may believe that everything is difficult for you. What do you then think happens in your brain? The more difficult you believe something is, the more that belief will be anchored in your unconscious, and the stronger it will become. And even in times when it's really easy, you'll say it's hard!

I remember very well the example of classic conditioning with Pavlov's dog during my courses of psychology at the University of Montreal. Pavlov rang a bell every time he gave food to his dog. At some point, Pavlov decided to ring the bell without serving food to the dog. Despite this, the dog still salivated. Pavlovian conditioning is thus a process by which the dog associates an already *programmed* response (saliva), which is normally triggered by a conditioned stimulus (the presence of food), with an *unconditioned* stimulus, such as the bell. That is to say that a neutral stimulus, which normally does not trigger any response (the sound of a bell), becomes a trigger. You understand that normally a dog does not salivate when listening to the sound of a bell.

It is the same with human beings! We have developed conditioned reflexes since childhood. For example, every time you try to do something, and you are told that it's difficult, and you're unable to do it, then you will be conditioned to see it as being difficult, and you surely will be unable to do it. You will no longer be able to see things that are easy, and that you are good or even excellent at doing! How can you change if you believe things are as hard as you think they are?

This false belief, "It's difficult, and I won't succeed," fuels your unconscious and becomes a habit! We must change this limiting belief into a dynamic belief. For example, start by changing what you tell yourself, into a positive and uplifting belief, such as "It's getting easier, and I'll get there!"

In the past, I learned a little trick to change my limiting beliefs into energizing beliefs, and it really works. You just have to find an elastic bracelet, one that does not cut the circulation or leave a mark on your skin. Every time you think the limiting belief of "it's hard…," slap yourself with the bracelet, and you'll change it into an energizing belief (Repeat it 3 times.).

This phenomenon makes you become more and more aware of what you say to yourself! By being conscious of what you say to yourself, it becomes easier making change and creating a new way of thinking and a new habit.

Your beliefs directly influence the way you act. If you say to yourself, "I can't do it," then you are right, and it is certain that you won't succeed. But if you say, "I'm going to make it happen," then surely, you'll get there, because you're going to condition your brain to do what is needed to get there (POWER OF POSITIVE THINKING)!

You will also create automations. It will be easier and easier for it to become automatic. For example, driving! In the beginning, when you learned to drive, you had to be focused on driving only. Now you can drive, listen to music, sing, and think of someone, all at the same time!

Keep in mind that a belief has the power to build you up or destroy you!

What if fear is part of your beliefs?

Do You Live According to Your Fears or Your Dreams?

Fear is very often a misperception of reality. It's often pertaining to something that has not yet happened! What are the types of fear? There are so many!!! Fear of rejection, fear of being criticized or humiliated, fear of failure, fear of public speaking, fear of travelling, fear of committing, fear of dying, self-doubt, and even fear of SUCCESS!!!

When you are afraid of something, your brain does not differentiate between the present and the future, or between the real and the imaginary. If, for example, you watch a horror movie, you are afraid even if it's unreal and imaginary!!! This proves that your brain does not differentiate between reality and imagination!!!

True fear, which deserves consideration and is quite normal, occurs when you face a real danger. For example, you meet a bear, or you are inside your house and it catches on fire!!! This fear is vital! It's a fear for survival!!!

Any fear you face (except the ones related to your survival), understand that it's only your imagination. Once you have overcome a fear, then you learn you are capable of doing so, and you can transcend that fear!

Focus on GAINS AND NOT LOSSES

Often, we will focus more on the losses than on gains, which is why we don't change. Know that for every change we make, there are losses and gains! It's inevitable!!!

For example, if you want to lose weight.

The losses could be:

- I will have to limit certain foods, such as high glycemic index foods, white bread, wheat pasta, chips, pastries, and fast food.
- I will have to limit the restaurants I go to.
- I will have to find time to do physical activities.

If you focus on these losses, you will keep your 10, 20, 30, 40, or 50 lbs. in excess, which may even increase with time!!!

If rather, you focus on the gains of liberating yourself of your excess weight.

Your winnings can be:

- I will have more energy and a feeling of well-being.
- I will improve my body's condition.
- My organs will work better.
- My blood pressure will decrease.
- My cholesterol level will drop.

- My heart rate will drop, and my heart will perform better.
- My sleep will improve.
- I'll be more focused.
- I will be able to be more present for my children and be a good example for them, who will imitate me in turn.
- I will leave to my children a beautiful legacy of values.
- I will feel more beautiful in my body.
- I will be an inspirational model for other people who also want to lose weight.

What do you think will happen if you focus on YOUR GAINS? WOW! You will surely succeed! It's a guarantee of success.

So, look at all these gains!!! Make a list!!! Post it in several places in your home.

This is truly an opportunity to grow and learn. We were designed to evolve! That is why we are human beings! We are programmed for change!!! Change must be part of us!

We are not on this earth to live a life in black and white.

We are made to live a MULTICOLOR life.

The *wheel of balance* is a powerful tool to determine YOUR goals!

This wheel features the 5 pillars for taking control of your health.

BODY
Physical Health
Nutrition/Supplementation
Physical Activity

MIND
Mental Health
Personal Development
Spirituality

SOCIETY
Intimate Relationships
Family Relationships
Friendship

FINANCES
Financial Situation
Career/Work

TOXIC OR NON-TOXIC ENVIRONMENT
Place in Which We Live

Start by situating your current position in each of the components. The center is the zero point (minimum limit) and the outside of the circle is 10 (maximum limit). For example, let's take your PHYSICAL HEALTH. On the line of PHYSICAL HEALTH, do you consider your physical health as a 0/10, 2/10 ... 5/10 (moderate), 8/10 or 10/10? Place a point on the line corresponding to that level. Be honest during this exercise. Then, do the same with all the other aspects. Gather the points with a colored pencil to see if your wheel is well balanced. Are there aspects of your life that deserve more attention?

Next, determine where you want to go, with a pencil of another color. What aspects do you want to focus more on? Also, write down the reasons why these aspects are important to you. The more reasons you have, the more you will be able to achieve your goals. Know that all these aspects are important, because they are all part of your GLOBAL HEALTH that will help you reach your OPTIMAL HEALTH!

Then, display those reasons and your goals at various strategic locations in your home, reminding and explaining the importance of you achieving them

By seeing them regularly, you will remain focused!

Wheel of balance

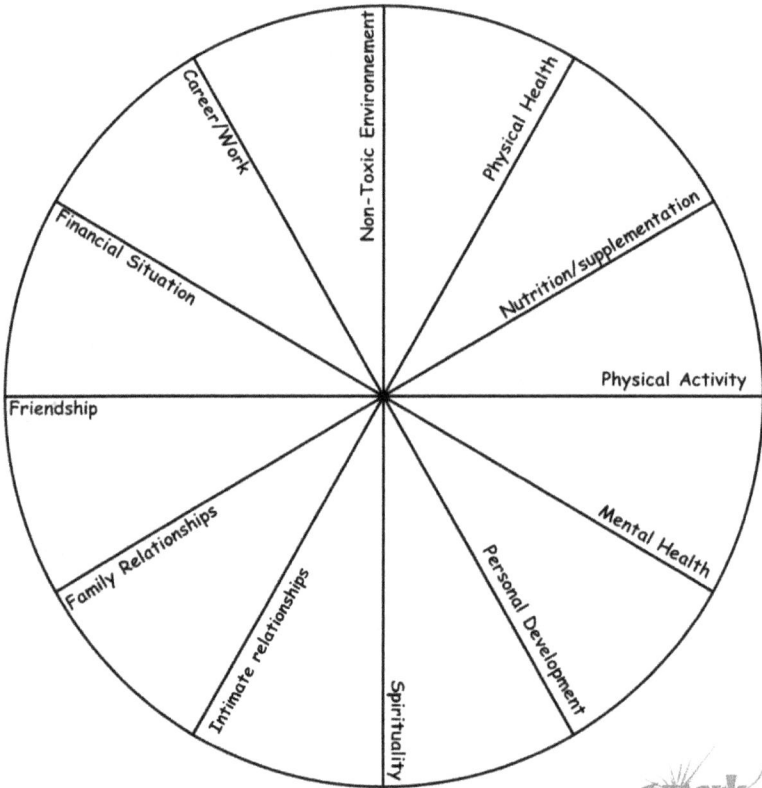

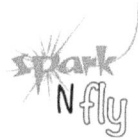

Now that you see with your own eyes the aspects of your life where you need to focus, we can help you by offering you the tools to achieve your goals.

Visit **Sparknflynow.com**

Pillar 3 :
SOCIETY

Chapter 8

DO YOUR RELATIONSHIPS FEED YOU?

Your relationships impact your mood, your physical well-being, and your mental health. With that in mind, it is key to ask yourself two critical questions about your relationships.

Do your relationships feed you, and do they allow you to exploit your full potential? This is key, because our relationships support us, nourish our souls, and provide the accountability we need to reach our dreams and goals. Without them, we would live in a void that would be unappealing and drab.

Up to now, we have focused on how you can achieve optimum health with the first two pillars: body and mind. These are really two very important pillars. I often put the emphasis on them, because without them, we can't achieve our best lives and our best selves. However, the 3rd pillar, SOCIETY is just as important!

The Impact of Your Relationships in Your Life

Do your relationships really impact your life? Do they allow you to achieve your goals? Without a shadow of a doubt, yes! The individuals you spend the most time with will either encourage or discourage you in reaching your goals and dreams. Finding your best self, and making the changes you want to make, requires individuals who are going to help you by being your cheerleaders, your accountability partners, but also a place to brainstorm and grow. Their influence can be key to the success or failure of your endeavors!

You know the expression, "You are the average of the 5 people around you?" Think about the people in your life and take the time to write down the names of the 5 people you spend the most time with. These may include your spouse, friends, boss, co-workers, sports partners, etc. Whoever they are, make sure that you have your 5 people before moving on to the next section.

Ask yourself these key questions about these 5 individuals. Be honest with yourself as you evaluate your connection with these individuals.

- Do these people, who have made the list, have an optimal level of energy and vitality?
- Do they take care of their physical, mental, emotional, and financial health?

What does your circle of success look like? Is it rather a circle that is destined for failure, to sabotage, stagnant, or dedicated to keep you from reaching your full potential? Will this circle help you to achieve your most important goals?

- What rating do you attribute to each of these 5 people? Be authentic!

Name: _____ = / 10
Name: _____ = / 10
Name: _____ = / 10
Name: _____ = / 10
Name: _____ = / 10

- Then, figure out the average of these 5 people, and you will have your grade!

___ + ___ + ___ + ___ + ___ =?
? / 5 = ___

Conclusion: If the average is 5/10, then you will be no more than a 5/10 person, because they will never assist in propelling you to the next level of your life. We inevitably end up looking like those people we spend the most time with. Nature is thus made that one merges with them on different domains. The question becomes, how can you make major changes to reach your optimal self, if you aren't surrounded by individuals who are trying to do the same?

If you want to optimize your health, then you will have to rub shoulders with individuals who give you an average of 8–9, or 10/10!

Surround yourself with people who:

- have found the path to optimal health;
- are aware of the 5 pillars to achieve optimum health;
- eat good, healthy, and energizing foods;
- have understood that supplementation of the highest quality has no price in our world today;
- know that sleep is primordial;
- train to profit from all the benefits of exercise;
- continue to grow in their personal development;
- and have chosen to take control of their health!

Follow **Sparknflynow.com**!!!

Create an environment that will turn you on and help you achieve your goals! Form a group that will elevate you to the highest peaks—not those that will extinguish the spark in you—your unique spark! A group is key, both for support and encouragement during moments when you seem to plateau, and to celebrate as you achieve your goals and dreams. These individuals can be making changes of their own, thus allowing you to support and encourage them as well.

If, for example, you want to lose weight:

- You will have to limit your time with people who are not physically active, who are obese, and who constantly nibble at low-quality restaurants, and eat fast foods.
- Find yourself a motivated companion who wants to change like you; or, better yet, who has already gone through the entire weight loss process and has succeeded. Follow him, train with him, and implement what tips you receive into your own lifestyle. This will motivate you, while at the same time, it will hold you accountable to someone else for creating change in your life.
- Find a coach, learn from a coach.
- Learn about nutrition and supplementation.
- Attend lectures and fill out your toolbox.
- Work on your personal growth so you do not lose sight of your goals.
- ESPECIALLY KEEP AWAY FROM THOSE WHO HAVE FAILED, AND MAY DISCOURAGE YOU!!! They dare not do what you do! It's just that simple! We call them Dream Breakers!

Personal growth is more than just achieving your goals. It is also understanding how you may be sabotaging yourself or allowing others to sabotage you. When you define who you want to be and how you want to live, there will be those around you who try to discourage you or convince you that it isn't possible to create change. They will tell you that the process is too big, and it is better to just accept your life how it is right now. As a result, they might get inside your head and get you to tell yourself the same things. Remember, they are not true! You can have the amazing health and life that you want. It is possible, but you have to make changes to stop the sabotage.

Now is the time to make a choice, using your average as a guide.

2 CHOICES are available to you:

1- You choose the status quo.
   (You stay with your average and make no changes.)

2- You change your environment to create the best version of yourself.
   (You increase your average to reach your full potential.)

You do not have to say goodbye to some people (like your family members, even if sometimes it would be for the best). However, spend much less time with them. You can even try to make them understand the situation. You never know, that could change these people and start them on their own journey to an optimal lifestyle!

Does Your Intimate Relationship Support You?

It is clear that for you to flourish, your spouse is very important. One of the priorities of any couple is to come together at the level of your values. Values are actually what is most important to you. They define you and how you interact with the larger world. If, for you, the respect value is a priority and not for your partner, then you will not be consistent with yourself in relation to your values in your relationship. You are likely to face regular disputes.

When two individuals can't agree on a shared value system that encourages and excites them both, that conflict will just continue to grow and create a situation unlikely to support growth and real change. Be honest with yourself. Is your relationship a source of support or a source of conflict? Are you both growing and changing for the better, or do you bring out the worst in each other?

It is important to establish rules as a couple, and a vision. Where are you going? Are you going in the same direction? Or are you both headed to two different destinations, with two completely different maps on how to get there?

One way to find out is through communication. This means more than just hearing the other person. It means being present, giving them your complete attention, and allowing them to express themselves fully. When you do so, you will make the connection deeper, and the understanding between the two of you will continue to grow.

Express what is important to you. You need to be willing to be open and honest with your partner about what gets you excited, what you feel passionate about, what hurts your feelings, what you appreciate, and what you want to change in yourself and your relationship. Do not think that your partner can guess everything. First and foremost, listen to what is important to your spouse. Always communicate constructively. Be genuine in the face of what you feel and live, while acknowledging the feelings and perceptions of your partner.

Know that man and woman are two beings and are very different. A man sees life in blue, with his blue glasses, and he hears with his blue hearing aids. As for a woman, she sees life in pink, with her pink glasses, and she hears with her pink hearing aids. These different perceptions can impact how each side reacts and how they choose to support or encourage each other. These differences can be a source of compromise and healing, or they can be a source of conflict. The key is communication.

In order to communicate, one must be able to fully understand the needs of the other. And for this, I recommend an excellent book that has changed my way of seeing the couple relationship: *Love and Respect*, by Dr. Emerson Eggerichs. This book helps you to better understand the needs of men and women, and how to communicate better. Personally, this is my favorite book that I have read in my lifetime! If, for you, the value LOVE is important, and it impacts the rest of the spheres of your life, then read this book. It can actually transform your relationship as a couple!

One of the keys to having a healthy relationship as a couple is having common projects. If one of your projects is to restore your health, then express it to your partner. Tell him your needs, how and why they are so important to you, and all the benefits that this could bring to you both. Express your motivations and reasons for doing so. If your partner does not want to follow you in the adventure towards health, but respects you and supports you positively, that's what is the most important. Then, seeing the results, he will probably follow you!

Relationships are based on genuine exchanges that nourish us, because we enter into a dynamic of mutual creation. In short, create your winning environment by surrounding yourself with extraordinary people who believe in you and who support you, whatever your goals are!

Pillar 4 : ENVIRONMENT

Chapter 9

THE INFLUENCE OF YOUR PHYSICAL ENVIRONMENT IN WHICH YOU LIVE

T he physical environment in which you live also affects your health. If you live in a polluted environment, it is clear that your health can really be impacted in a negative way.

Degenerative diseases (cancer, cardiovascular diseases, respiratory diseases, stroke, diabetes, autoimmune diseases, etc.) are continuing to increase, and these diseases continue to become more aggressive. It is now said that almost one in two people will have cancer in their lifetime. What do we foresee for the future? Will this statistic increase again and again? The future looks grim, as our environment is being poisoned. The environment in which we live is no longer that of the past.

Did you know that around 143,000 chemicals have been listed worldwide, according to an analysis carried out under the REACH regulations of the European Union[26]?

The number of chemicals we are exposed to on a daily basis is astounding. We find them in all the products we use on a daily basis, from cleaning ourselves to cleaning our homes. Even the materials used to build our homes carry chemical loads, which are passed onto our homes. Those chemicals become part of our bodies, as our exposure continues. However, it can be more damaging, the longer the exposure.

I invite you to consult the *Report on Toxic Substances Detected in Blood from the Umbilical Cord of Newborns in Canada.*

Go to **sparknflynow.com** (skin-health section) to access the link.

The burden of the toxic products that Canadians carry in them, without even knowing it, is revealing. We also need to be worried about the fate of our children, as already around 100 chemical substances have been detected in the umbilical cord blood of children being born. What are some of the chemicals being found?

Heavy metals, endocrine disruptors, and carcinogenic substances, such as:

- DIOXINS AND FURANS
- EDP (polybrominated diphenyl ethers)
- CFC-14 (tetrafluoromethanes)
- ORGANOCHLORATED PESTICIDES

- METHYLMERCURE
- LEAD
- PCBs (polychlorinated biphenyls)
- And more…

What are the cumulative and synergistic effects of these chemicals? What is the lifetime impact of these toxic chemicals on your environment and your body?

Worrisome? Yes, there is something to worry about!

Imagine if, from birth, we were already contaminated by all these chemicals! What is the impact of this on our development? This is exactly what is happening to our children today. The impact of the chemicals they are exposed to today, and carry in their bodies, can change their development.

That is why I am directing you to reflect on the importance of your environment, especially the need for you to exercise the ability to choose good antioxidants, which can greatly help you in protecting yourself from some of these dangerous oxidants (free radicals) impacting your health and that of your children.

What Does the Water You Drink Each Day Contain?

Today's water is no longer the water we had several years ago. The changes reflect how our environment has been altered, which is impacting our health.

Water analyses note the presence of a variety of chemical substances, such as:

- Antibiotics
- Hormones
- Heavy metals
- Petroleum and petroleum products
- Bacteria and living microorganisms
- Plastics and cosmetics
- Etc.

This is just the beginning. Depending on the source, the amount of chemicals can be substantially higher. Pipes can degrade, adding high levels of lead into the water, which can have impacts on the health and development of children. It has been discovered that brain damage can be significant with lead exposure. Yet this is just one issue facing individuals every time they turn on the tap.

In fact, authorities have determined what they deem is the safe level of chemical exposure. The Canadian and U.S. governments allow a certain amount of chemicals in our water. They also use filtration systems, which use chemicals to eradicate germs or harmful substances from the water, putting these chemicals into the water supply.

So you drink water from the tap that is not free of chemicals. It can affect your health, because it is not pure.

You might be thinking: "That's why I don't drink tap water. I make it a regular part of grocery shopping to pick up bottled water. It is the healthier option." Do you think bottled spring water is better than tap? Warning: that is not the case!

This source of water is mostly available in plastic bottles, which are made from chemicals. Those chemicals can leak from the plastic into the water. It seems that it is mainly the endocrine disrupters potentially released by plastic bottles that have caught the attention of toxicologists in recent years.

Endocrine disruptors are those substances that disrupt the proper functioning of our hormones, either by imitating them or preventing them from doing their job. Phthalates and Bisphenol A (BPA), two families of chemical agents used in the manufacturing of several plastics, have a configuration similar to hormones. What about other types of plastic?

Is surface water or artesian well water any better? I recommend that you have it analyzed, as it can also contain an exhaustive amount of heavy metals and other substances that can harm your health. Many companies analyze your water cheaply, or even free of charge, so why not? Recognize that just because it has fancy packaging and great marketing slogans on it, doesn't mean that it is going to be a quality option.

What about filtered water? With filtered water, the water is cleared of its chlorine taste, but still the majority of the harmful substances pass through the filter. It means that you are drinking the chemicals and substances you thought were taken out.

Have you heard of distilled water? The distillation makes it possible to obtain perfectly pure water. In the case of distilled water, it is a demineralized water, completely free of toxins, but also of minerals (organic and inorganic). According to some water's specialists, this is not the best choice, because you are drinking water that has the good stripped from it.

What types of water are the best choice for you to get the benefits of water, without the additional chemical load?

According to the SANOVIV Medical Institute, water filtered by reverse osmosis is the best option. The high-quality osmosis filters are effective and provide excellent water, by stripping out the chemicals and negative aspects. Reverse osmosis is a water purification system containing substances in solution by using a very fine filtering system, which allows only water molecules to pass. An osmosed water is cleared of chlorine, and also metals and residues, as well as organic and inorganic matter. It is characterized by its total absence of taste.

In the case of distilled and osmosed water, it may be necessary to re-mineralize it to obtain more alkaline water, which is beneficial for the body's pH balance. It is easy to add a mineral cartridge to the osmosis filtration system, which can be installed in your home. Personally, I have a reverse osmosis system (installed under my sink), and I have clearly noticed the difference and enjoyed the benefits of this water.

Are You Actually Safe in Your Own Home?

The majority of home care and cleaning products are toxic. When you mostly use mainstream cleaning products, they often include a warning about how to use them with protective gloves, and to avoid contact with your skin or eyes. Yet this residue is what we are leaving behind on the surfaces and items within our homes.

These products are so harmful that they cannot be swallowed, breathed, or touched.

Many display all different types of symbols, such as:

• the skull and cross bone
• danger
• irritation
• danger of poisoning
• flammable
and more.

Have you already listed all the cleaning and maintenance products in your home? Here are just a few that I came up with.

Cleaning products for:

- All-purpose
- Degrease
- Sinks and counters
- Scour cooking surfaces
- Oven
- Dishes and dishwasher
- Hands
- Windows
- Toilet bowls and toilets
- Baths and showers
- Furniture
- Wood
- Ceramic
- Floors
- Walls
- Stainless steel
- Clothing (dry cleaning, laundry detergent, bleach, and spot removers)

This is just the beginning. Here are a few more potential options:

- Anti-static products
- Softeners (liquids and sheets)
- Odor control products
- In diffuser and aerosol
- Carpet cleaner and deodorizer
- Protection products
- For fabrics, leather, and wood
- Disinfecting products

- Piping products
- Solvents for molds

As you can see, the list can include multiple products, based on where you live, the type of furniture and appliances that you own, and the type of maintenance or cleaning you have to accomplish in a typical day or week.

It's amazing to see the incredible amount of toxins that emit toxic odors, which float in your environment to smother you overtime and negatively impact your health. What do you think?

You would be surprised to learn about all the chemical substances that are contained in all these products! If you accumulate them, you will have an exhaustive list of carcinogens harmful to your health, as well as that of your children, and even your pets!

Why Get Intoxicated When There Are Natural Solutions for Multiple Uses?

Why not use what nature has given us? I suggest you read the book, *The Healthy Home*, written by Dr. Myron Wentz and Dave Wentz, to learn natural cleansing solutions.

Distilled white vinegar is a mild acid that easily dissolves soap residues, cleans glass, disinfects surfaces, and is a perfect fabric softener.

Lemon juice is a mild acid with slight bleach properties. It helps to remove stains and restore whites to white. A little lemon juice squeezed, and the job is done! Lemon juice can also be used to clean rust, soap scum, and stains caused by water.

Here are some examples that you can use from the book, *The Healthy Home*.

For an all-purpose cleaner:
* One liter of warm water, 4 tablespoons of baking soda, and 1 teaspoon of vinegar.

To clean your windows:
* 3 cups water, ¼ cup white vinegar, and 1 ½ tablespoons lemon juice.

To eliminate odors:
* Put a few drops of essential lemon, orange, or eucalyptus oil into the water, and spray in your home.

To replace clothes softener:
* ½ cup white vinegar in the washer to soften the clothes and remove the static.

These home solutions are simple, effective, and inexpensive, and do not affect your health, or that of your children or your pets.

What Do You Put on Your Skin?

We talked about the chemicals that are contained in the environment in which we live. What about the body care products that you put on your skin? We greatly underestimate the chemicals in skin care products. Have you ever tried to read the labels? Did you manage to understand? What do you think of this exhaustive list?

You probably know about transdermal patches used by people trying to quit smoking. They deliver a nicotine dosage that penetrates the skin and finds its way into the bloodstream. It's the same with all the products you put on your skin. They penetrate the layers of the skin, ending up in your blood; thus, they can greatly disrupt your health.

If you are not ready to eat what you put on your skin, then do not put it on!

How many body care products do you use per day? It will amaze you how much of a chemical load you are adding to your organism. Making adjustments in this area is key to changing the amount of chemicals that your body and systems are exposed to on a daily basis.

- Toothpaste
- Mouthwash
- Flossing
- Facial Cleaner

- Cleansing
- Toning
- Day cream
- Night Cream
- Serum
- Eye contour
- Masks
- Deodorant
- Antiperspirant
- Shampoo
- Conditioner
- Soap
- Shower Gel
- Shaving foam
- Hair removal cream
- Mascara
- Face powder
- Lipstick
- Eyeliner
- Hair styling gel
- Foam
- Hairspray
- Nail polish
- Fragrance
- Perfume
- Sunscreen
- After-sun lotion
- Anti-mosquito lotion
- Toilet paper
- Hygienic Tampons
- Wipes
- Dressings

All these products contain a phenomenal list of harmful ingredients that represent a real danger to your health (nitrosamine, lead, heavy metals, parabens, phthalates, hydroquinone, 1,4-dioxan), just to name a few. By counting all the ingredients found in all of the products you have used, you would be terrified! Imagine how hard your emunctory organs (which eliminate waste) have to work to eliminate all this from your body and manage the chemical load from all the chemicals you are exposed to during a typical day.

How is it then that these chemicals, which are so harmful, are allowed to be used in these products? Do the authorities really care about our health? It's up to you to decide! Your skin represents the largest organ in your body. It is your first barrier against the outside world, protecting you from chemicals.

Every month, you completely regenerate the outer layer of your skin. However, your skin is porous, so you still need to be aware of what you are being exposed to on a daily basis. Your skin cells are constantly attacked and damaged by free radicals (pollution; chemicals in water, earth, and air; cigarettes, preservatives, stress, etc.), and they must constantly defend themselves with strong weapons. It only takes a few minutes for the free radicals to end up in the blood and create damage, which is sometimes unrecoverable.

One study found that the umbilical cord of newborns contained a variety of chemicals absorbed by the mother during pregnancy. ENVIRONMENTAL DEFENCE tested the umbilical cord blood of three newborn babies and found each child was born with 55 to 121 toxic compounds and possible cancer-causing chemicals in their bodies. Of the 137 chemicals found in total, 132 are reported to cause cancer in humans or animals, 110 are considered toxic to the brain and nervous system, and 133 cause developmental and reproductive problems in mammals[27].

This little being is so fragile, is not yet in this world, and must endure all these toxins being given to him via the umbilical cord of the mother. He is born pre-polluted!

You can download the PRE-NATAL POLLUTION report on **Sparknflynow.com**.

The skin:

- is the largest of all our organs
- has a protective and thermoregulatory function
- is a powerful vehicle for the elimination of our toxins
- is a reflection of what is happening inside our body
- is directly related to effective liver detoxification
- is the expression of our physical and emotional state

Several elements have an impact on the state of the skin, hair, and nails: diet, hydration, smoking, drugs, stress, sleep, digestion, pollution, irritants, alcohol and drugs, hormones, diseases, and more.

It is very important to use body care products that are trustworthy: free of parabens, parabens derivatives, and harmful chemicals. The ingredients must be free from toxins and contaminants. The mention of *Bio* or a *natural product* is not a pledge of purity. Beware and learn!

Additionally, feeding and protecting your skin externally is not enough, as it also needs to be nourished internally with minerals, vitamins, phytonutrients, and antioxidants that are essential nutrients for health. Vitamins, including antioxidants, will help neutralize some of the free radicals that penetrate your skin. Good fats, such as Omega 3, are also essential to repair the skin, moisturize it, and give it flexibility.

If you have skin and hair problems, they can be related to nutritional deficiencies, nutrient assimilation, and a troubled digestive system. It's the reflection of your interior! Instead of applying a multitude of products to your skin, think of feeding your interior!

We invite you to visit the **HEALTH-BEAUTY Skin Program,** at sparknflynow.com, for access to a range of products free of toxins, parabens, and paraben derivatives. Try it, and you will never want to apply anything else on your precious skin. It may also be necessary to detoxify your emunctory organs to eliminate your accumulated toxins (chemicals and additives in your environment).

You can also visit the **Detox Program** at sparknflynow.com.

In sum, the environment in which you live is one of the most important pillars in achieving optimal health. As much as possible, minimize contact with chemicals, whether external or internal, and protect yourself by consuming the highest quality antioxidants, vitamins, phytonutrients, and minerals.

The skin needs to be NOURISHED, PROTECTED, and RENEWED optimally!

---

[26] Tortorello, M. (2012, March 14). Is It Safe to Play Yet? Going to Extreme Lengths to Purge Household Toxins. The New York Times. (From report PRE POLLUTED : JUNE 2013).
[27] PRE-POLLUTED : A Report on Toxic Substances Detected in Blood from the Umbilical Cord of Newborns in Canada, June 2013.

Pillar 5 :
FINANCES

Chapter 10

THE IMPACT OF YOUR FINANCES ON YOUR HEALTH

People's Top 3 Concerns (Health, Money, and Time)

I t is a fact that physical health, whether yours or your loved ones, your financial situation, and the time you spend on yourself and your family are the three most important concerns of the majority of people. So far, we have talked a lot about physical health. Now I would like to focus on people's concern about money and their financial health.

Many people experience stress because their finances are deficient. Yes, I did say deficient, since it can make you stressed or even physically ill. Think about the last time you had concerns about money. Worrying about it likely made your stomach knot up and brought on other physical symptoms. These are the physical signs from your mental stress. Yet it would probably surprise you to know that your beliefs about money could be leading to your financial struggles.

Since our childhood, false limiting beliefs about money have been inserted into our brains. Yes, I say limitative, because they slow down our full potential as an individual and bring us unfounded fears that can keep us from acting in a way that allows us to reach our full potential. Here are just a few of the sayings that you might have heard growing up:

- "Money cannot buy happiness."
- "We do not need money to be happy."
- "Money is dirty; it's bad; it's unhealthy."
- "Money ...

But are any of these statements really accurate? Most of these statements focus on the negative aspects of money and can influence your financial worth, but for those looking to make changes in their lifestyle and pursue their passions, how they view money needs to change as well. Those without money find themselves limited in their ability to access better food options, better physical opportunities, and more.

Never forget that it is our childhood that is the basis of our internal construction. It is then nourished by all our various experiences, into childhood and adulthood. Our beliefs are anchored as habits and can be very difficult to change. At the same time, our perceptions of the world around us are often shaped to reinforce our beliefs. We can often miss out on opportunities because we allow our beliefs to limit our point of view and shape our experiences.

How can you change your beliefs? It involves going further into your thought process and asking yourself why you believe things are a certain way. Then, ask yourself if that belief is serving you or limiting you from taking the next step to reaching your goals. Your beliefs could be one of your greatest obstacles to creating a healthy lifestyle for you and your family.

Realizing all of this gives you power! The power to create change and spark a healthy lifestyle—mentally, emotionally, physically, and financially.

Money is, in fact, a means of acquiring freedom: seeing children and grandchildren grow up, spoiling them when you want to, taking vacations, eating organic foods and extra-fresh products, taking care of yourself by using osteopathy, massage therapy, acupuncture, and chiropractic, and so on. It also affords you the ability to provide cell micro-nutrition of the highest quality, to alter today's nutritional deficiencies and protect yourself from degenerative diseases and premature aging. Why not use money to fulfill our passions that stimulate us and give us energy? Even more, to discover this magnificent planet that deserves to be visited in all its little nicks and corners! What would you think if we considered money as a factor of opportunity, instead of a detriment or a negative?

Money gives us the power to create, to create a life in our image, the life that we have always imagined! Money can finance our dreams. It allows us to become what we desire the most, and gives us the ability to pursue our passions. It can also provide a better future for our children. For example, paying so they may attend university or a private school, because education is something you view as necessary for their well-being.

What do you think? Would this way of thinking about money be much closer to your values and your reality? Undoubtedly!

Finally, being financially free means being emotionally and spiritually free! It means not worrying about the end of each month, because we know that we have financial freedom. This freedom allows us to direct our energies towards what excites us and makes us feel alive!

It's sad having to abandon a dream because of a lack of funds. It would be unfortunate to have to opt out of private schools for our children, simply because we do not have the means to send them. Also, there are the experiences and traveling that we would miss out on because it is financially out of our reach. For example, not taking our children to Walt Disney because our finances won't allow it. How would we feel in these moments? Life is short, and you only have one, so there is no place for regret and "I should have…but I didn't have the means."

Money is a great tool to help you make your life what you always hoped it would be! You need to alter your perceptions of money in order to nurture your dreams and, above all, to realize them!

All this has nothing to do with luck. We become proactive in the process of creating our lives. We create it in our image and according to the beliefs that inhabit us. If our beliefs are limiting, our lives will also be limiting, and we will not be able to reach our full potential. The possibilities are endless if our beliefs are energizing and enriching, and we take the necessary actions to attain them.

Not realizing our dreams is like slowly dying, wishing for something different without acting on it.

Take the time to ask yourself the following questions:

- What has become of your dreams?
- Does your financial situation affect your dreams?
- Are you unable to see the big picture because your financial situation does not permit you to?

Here is a list of people's greatest dreams:

- Paying off their debts
- Travelling
- Having more vacation time and being able to live freely
- Spoiling their spouses and children, making sure they are fulfilled
- Having a passionate job
- Being healthy by eating high quality and organic products
- Offering ourselves pure, effective, and high-quality supplements
- Having a family doctor in a private clinic

- Preparing a magnificent retirement
- Owning the house of their dreams
- Owning the car of their dreams
- Leaving an inheritance

What has become of your dreams? Are you actually building them, or are you missing out on your life, your one and only life?

It is time for empowerment and leaving our mark on this earth! Our lives deserve to be fully lived!

By eliminating your limiting beliefs, and discovering how money is your friend, you can move forward, claiming a different relationship with money and your finances. Everyone knows the saying, "Do not put all your eggs in one basket." Now, let us explore the difference between active and passive income.

Passive Income : A Jewel of the Economy

First, it is important to differentiate between active and passive income. Active income is an inflow of money from the sale of any product or service. This income depends entirely on you. For example, if you are an employee in a company, every hour worked will give you an amount of money. You work 40 hours, so you get paid for your 40 hours. You exchange your time for money. You may be self-employed, or an entrepreneur. It's the same thing; you exchange, once again, hours (your time) for money. In either case, if you stop your business, your earnings will cease completely.

So, you have to be active to raise money. That's why it's active income.

- I work (active) = I earn $
- I do not work (not active) = I do not earn $

It is now clear that with active income, you should never stop to continue to receive money.

- What happens if you have to stop working?
- What happens if you are sick, or your children or spouse are sick, and you have to stop working in the short, medium, or long term?

There is no more money coming in, since you have to be active and present to collect the money.

- Yes, you can have a few paid sick days a year.
- Yes, you may have unemployment benefits, but your salary is drastically reduced.
- Yes, you may have private insurance, but it may only cover you over a specific period; will it cover you throughout your illness? Your lifestyle will probably be reduced.

Now, what about *passive income*, considered one of the jewels of the economy? Passive income, unlike active income, does not depend entirely on us. It is not proportional to the time and effort spent on the income-generating task. It derives its strength from the automation of tasks rather than from repetition. It may take longer to set up at the beginning—a phase in which it does not generate much income. On the other hand, it demands less effort, and can generate revenues 24/7. Once in place, it requires very little or no active participation on our part, which means we earn money even when we are away. It does not require our physical presence; we can be on the other end of the planet on a beautiful beach, and the income will continue to accumulate!

It is possible to have an active income while working to build a passive income, until the day your passive income becomes more important than your active income! We can then decide whether or not to leave our active income.

What types of passive income can we invest in?
1. Real estate (rental homes, cottages, condos, apartments, etc.)
2. Write a book (however, you must have talent, time, and inspiration!)
3. Making a music CD, or singing (again, there must be talent and, often, contacts in the music industry)
4. Investments in the stock market
5. Low risk investments

Maybe there is nothing in all this that interests you. What other passive income is there?

Network marketing has thought of you!

There is no need for any qualifications or diplomas. The only need is to enjoy connecting with people. If you want to impact their lives, this is a great way to work without ever really working.

Network marketing does not require any infra-structure, and its startup cost is very low. It is the opportunity to have the benefits of the self-employed worker (possibility to deduct expenses on taxes: mortgage or rent, home and auto insurance, heating and electricity, telephone, cellular, and internet; car: rental, repair, petrol, licenses, and registration; training, events, congress, and travels; books and stationery; computer; work accessories; etc.).

It is also the possibility of working alone or in a team. However, the strength of network marketing is teamwork. The more we help others, the more we receive. Instead of focusing on the weaknesses of people, we focus on strengths. We are joining our forces. It is an extraordinary way to transform and evolve as a human being.

Now, when you understand the power and benefits of network (relational) marketing, the focus must be on what we are interested in, and on the following question: Does it really respond to a need for the society?

If so, we must continue the process, since we want network marketing that will persist over time. It will thus ensure the long-term security of what we will create.

- Is the product or service offered of the highest quality?
- Does the company offer exceptional products that meet current and future needs?

Since you do not want the company to cease doing business in 2 years, and you do not want everything to collapse:

- Does the company have an exemplary past?
- Is the CEO exemplary and integral?
- Does the company's vision and mission align with our values?
- Has the company made any progress in research and technology over the years, and continues to progress?

These are many questions to look for when choosing the one that will align with our values. Maybe we do not have any knowledge in the field, but if we carry an interest, and we understand the need, and we have the desire to learn, then it's for us.

Do you think that this is not for you? If that's the case, then look at the other types of passive revenues that are available to you and that I shared with you, and understand that this type of income is, in my view, a necessity to ensure security in this uncertain world.

The network marketing and direct sales profession hit a new record high in 2015, with 183.7 billion dollars in global sales[28]. It is recognized and legal. It is taught in certain universities. It is considered by several wealthy people, including Robert Kiyosaki, author of several successful books, including *Rich Dad, Poor Dad*, as the enterprise of the 21st century.

The *conventional* company is moving towards 100% of your own efforts. *Network marketing* is oriented towards the following statement: "It is better to have 1% of the efforts of 100 people, than 100% of your own efforts." This corresponds much more to the values of mutual help, sharing, nurturing, teamwork, community, and excellence.

If you want to know more about it, since it is much more in line with your values, then I invite you to contact: sparknflynow@gmail.com. With all that I have shared with you in this chapter, you now understand that physical and financial health are closely linked. It is important to ensure financial security.

Money allows you to better take care of your physical health, and your physical health allows you to better enjoy your money.

Have you ever wondered about what you would like to HAVE, DO, and BE? Here is a very interesting exercise[29]! See great things in your future! No limits!

1- If you had all the time, money, and health ...

- What would you have that you do not have?
- What would you do that you do not?
- What would you be that you are not?

* In each circle, write down your HAVE, DO, and BE.

Have

Do

Be

2 - What would be the annual cost that would allow you to offer all this? Do not be afraid!

_____ $

3 - If you continue doing what you do for 5 years, do you think you will achieve this lifestyle?

Yes   No

If you checked YES to question 3, then congratulations! You probably have multiple sources of PASSIVE income! You must be well supported!

If you checked NO, then you have to do something. Do not limit yourself to the minimum. Make yourself financially and physically healthy!

We are ready to accompany you in this process of creating passive income. You can contact me at: sparknflynow@gmail.com.

I have shared a lot of information about key areas that you need to address to achieve optimal health and the best life possible for you! Still, the only way to get there is with help. You need a support system to create these changes. That is where a coach comes in. Next, I will discuss the importance of a coach in your journey to optimal health!

---

[28] Source: WFDSA.org

[29] Thanks for my friend, Serge Deslonchamps, who is the creator of this exercise.

Chapter 11

WHY HAVE A COACH TO SUCCEED?

A coach serves to accompany and guide you to real change. As you saw in Chapter 7, change scares many people. If that's your case, you're normal! Do not forget that fear is not even reality. You anticipate things that have not even happened, and it blocks your ability to take action. Recognize that those fears are there, and surround yourself with people who believe in you, to help you to push through those fears, instead of allowing them to paralyze you.

However, that is not enough. You will also require a coach, a person who can guide you and help put you back on track when needed. After all, no one makes a change without a few setbacks. A coach can motivate you to pick yourself up and keep moving forward.

The coach lights the way for you, providing a map to follow toward your goals and dreams. Coaching opens the way toward achieving your objectives because, very often, you won't see the obstacles and challenges in your path until you are right on top of them.

Why is that the case?

As you create change in your life, you also experience changing emotions that can disrupt your logical thinking and make you completely forget where you should be headed. Your emotions can make you relive experiences from your past and completely lose sight of your objectives. How can this happen? Because you get so focused on the past, you lose the ability to focus on the only part of your life that you can control, which is the moment you are in right now!

Have you heard the expression, *"Eating your emotions?"* Often, people who act in this way do not become aware of the impact of this behavior until it is too late. By then, it has become an unconscious habit, with negative consequences. You have to find the right balance between your emotions and your logic. When you are too focused on your emotions, you are no longer able to apply your logic and reasoning to the circumstances and situations you face.

A coach serves as a guide to constantly steer you back towards your goals. A coach guides you by offering you a framework, know-how, clarification, an attentive ear, and realistic solutions. Unlike a psychologist, who turns to the problem (childhood and past), the coach focuses on the *now*, and the solutions that you can create and embrace. You want results NOW!

That's the approach I use myself when coaching people!

How many coaches should you have? Good question! You can have one for each area: a coach for nutrition and supplementation needs, a coach for physical activity, and a professional coach to take your career to the next level. Most coaches are specialized, but some are able to provide expertise in several areas.

The point is to find the coach or coaches for the changes you want to make in your life, based on the areas that you have identified as needing improvement.

However, in my opinion, the most important aspects for getting started are your physical and mental health. Invest first here! Your health is priceless, and when you lose it, you lose everything else.

The first coach you need to look for is one who can guide you through the process of healthier eating, finding the right supplements, and getting your body into its optimal state. Doing so will allow you to bring your mental and emotional health back in balance as well. Then you can start turning your life into one that allows you to pursue your passion and your life's purpose.

Every human being needs to have a guide, to have outside help to stay on track to achieve their goals. You can see it when you look at a top athlete. He didn't get to the top of his sport without assistance from others. Who did he rely on to help him achieve his goals?

He surrounded himself with the best to achieve his goals. His path means the best trainers, the best coaches, and the best equipment. He gives his body the best food and supplements to build up his energy and muscles, and to put his body on the path to optimal performance. The more he climbs to his biggest goal, the more he will have to readjust, and perhaps even change his coaches, to go to a higher level. I know this personally since I have been a world-class athlete myself.

It's the same for you! Choose coaches to assist you in reaching your goals. But once you achieve them, then don't be afraid to change coaches in order to attain the next level.

1- Do you really want to reach your goal?
2- Is it truly important to you?
3- Is it really worth it?
4- Are you ready to give up on it?

If you answered this way, then you need to take the next step.

1- Yes
2- Yes
3- Yes
4- No

To ensure your success, and not waste your time, invest in yourself by getting a coach!

The coach will help you carve out a new path to follow in your life's journey. With the help of a coach, you can gain the skills and knowledge necessary to set the milestones that will enable you to achieve your goals and create an amazing life!

How can you choose the right coach for yourself? Find out what they focus on and their areas of expertise. You might find that you need more than one coach, based on the areas of your life where you want to create real change. It might start out with your health and physical well-being, but don't feel that you have to stop there!

Mentors and coaches are a great way to keep you moving forward and creating the best life for yourself. The best part is that you can be a positive impact on others in your life, including your family and friends. Creating real and meaningful change starts with you!

The coach will help you recreate yourself.

The only day that exists is TODAY!

Do not wait until tomorrow; tomorrow, you will find another excuse not to do it.

Every human being should dream BIG. Every human being deserves to live an AMAZING life! However, that amazing life can't happen if you aren't giving your body and mind everything it needs to create optimal health. To make the best choices for your health, you need to understand how everything is interconnected and works together toward success.

My mission is to help you make better choices to bring you to true health. You will discover what it is like to live a life ENERGIZED and STIMULATING! It comes about through global health.

My LIFE VISION is TO CREATE an EPIDEMIC of HEALTHY PEOPLE around the world!

I want you to build the best life for yourself!

If you want to develop your health at every level, starting first with your physical and mental health, I invite you to discover this great movement at Sparknflynow.com.

Never forget that knowledge gives you power! The more knowledge you have, the better the life that you can create for yourself. May you take the steps to Spark N Fly, and join the movement for optimal health!

Isabelle Paquette
Creator of the great movement, Spark N Fly

About the Author

Isabelle Paquette is the author of *Spark N Fly, The 5 Pillars for Taking Control of Your Health* and the creator of the movement of the same name. She is a health professional determined to create a movement of global health by educating people about what they must choose to nourish their bodies and improve other aspects of their lives. In addition, she is an osteopath, naturopath, and speaker, who works with individuals to optimize their health, both physically and mentally. Isabelle had first embarked on a career as a physiotherapist, a career she practiced for eleven years during which she began studying osteopathy and decided to add naturopathy. She is an osteopath, graduated from the Centre Ostéopathique du Québec (COQ) and a naturopath, in addition to being a nutrition consultant certified by the Sanoviv Medical Institute.

That's not all! She also holds a major in psychology from the University of Montreal and also has a great experience in the field of sports competition since she was previously a world-class athlete in Taekwondo (5th in the world) and an instructor in this same sport. In addition, concerned to share her knowledge on health, she is a speaker who is dedicated to optimizing the physical and mental health of anyone concerned about her well-being.

Her work also includes coaching and mentoring individuals looking to create meaningful change in their lives through changes in their health, wealth, and goals. Isabelle assists individuals in their journey to true health by offering them the route and tools needed to achieve this.

Her conviction to *create* an epidemic of healthy people came after an event that disrupted her life in 2014: **her former life partner's colorectal cancer.** Her story is extraordinary, miraculous, and deserves to be heard. Isabelle sincerely believes that every person has in themselves the *Spark*, and SPARK N FLY movement has been designed to help you on your voyage to a lifestyle centered on true health.

Would you like a LIFE where you live fully and intensely, where you have energy, vitality, and optimal health? If you would like to know how she does it, then read this book. It can truly improve your life!

THE VISION OF SPARK N FLY is to CREATE AN EPIDEMIC OF HEALTHY PEOPLE WORLDWIDE!

Join the SPARK N FLY movement!
www.sparknflynow.com

You have just discovered the importance of
TAKING CONTROL of your health.

To follow up on your reading,
I suggest you visit my website:
sparknflynow.com

I have designed several programs
to optimize your health.